Roderick Lane's interest in na[...] mother, a hospital matron who took an unconventional line with patients – opting for natural remedies rather than drugs. He went on to study Chinese medicine as part of his Martial Arts training in the 1970s.

Roderick was lecturer in Clinical Nutrition at Howell College from 1990 to 1993 and Secretary of the National Guild of Clinical Nutritionists from 1988 to 1992. He also co-founded the London College of Naturopathic Medicine and Health Science in 1992, and has since filled the post of Registrar of the College and lectures in Clinical Nutrition and Protocol.

Now practising at the Eden Medical Centre in London, he holds Diplomas in Clinical Nutrition, Holistic Health and Naturopathy. Among his patients was the late Princess of Wales.

Sarah Stacey is an award-winning journalist, specialising in health, beauty and gardening, a TV producer and bestselling author. She is currently Wellbeing Editor on the *Mail on Sunday YOU magazine*.

She has worked on most of the leading UK newspapers, including the *Daily Telegraph*, *Financial Times* and *The Sunday Times*. She has also been Beauty and Health Editor on the *Telegraph magazine*, Executive Health and Beauty Editor on the *Daily Express* and Health Editor on *Harpers & Queen*.

Sarah was elected first Honorary Chair of the Guild of Health Writers in 1994 and in 1997 co-founded the Food Labelling AGenda (FLAG).

Sarah has extensive experience of local, national and international radio and television broadcasting, and has reported for BBC's *Watchdog*. Her two most recent books *The Beauty Bible* and *Feel Fabulous Forever*, co-written with Josephine Fairley, are both international bestsellers.

# Praise for *The Adam & Eve Diet*

**Terence Stamp**, actor:

'I wish Roderick Lane's system had been around in 1968 when I was taking tentative steps to heal myself. His insights on diet and nutrition are some of the most relevant I have discovered. In a world where we are beginning to understand that each one of us should take responsibility for our own health, this book is a sound step in the right direction.'

**Dr Robert Cass**, naturopathic physician and chiropractor, Atlanta, Georgia:

'Dr Roderick Lane's contribution to the overwhelming and often confusing volumes of information in the field of clinical nutrition comes as a very welcome breath of fresh air. His clear and specific approach cuts through the complexities of this powerfully emerging science with suggestions and protocols that are revealing of Dr Lane's many years of successful practice. This work will quickly feature high in the list of "must have" books on the healing arts, in professional and public libraries alike. Dr Lane is to be congratulated for this great addition to the information base.'

**Kenneth Fish**, DC, Director The Wellsprings Clinic, Maryland:

'I first spoke with Dr Lane in 1996, when he was kind enough to consult with me regarding nutritional support for Lupus patients. Dr Lane has exceptional insight into the endocrine and nutritional aspects of health and healing, and I have turned to him for advice in treating some of my more difficult cases.

I have personally followed Dr Lane's advice for my own health problems. As a result, my weight is now under control, I have more energy and feel better that I have in years. I highly recommend him to readers everywhere who may have tried other nutritional approaches without success. This may well be the key to your better health and quality of life.'

**Jane Upton**, 42, management consultant:

'I feel passionately supportive of this nutritional system because I felt so dreadful when I first went to Roderick Lane in 1994. I had been tired and generally unwell for a long time but my doctor had just said it was stress. Roderick said that I had a sugar problem and prescribed a diet to help. I got better little by little but today I am very fit and I have a greater understanding about my body and the way it works and what it needs.'

**Janie Romer**, 45, singer songwriter and mother of two:

'After a misspent youth I had two children and turned into an earth mother. After five years my body was exhausted and I could barely walk upstairs. Within three days of going on Roderick Lane's diet, and taking the supplements he suggested, I remembered what it was like to be more alive. After a few weeks, I had whittled down a dress size and I had so much more energy. I began to exercise again and I could run from A to B instead of dragging myself. Ending the cycle of exhaustion and craving (and the guilt that goes with that) opens so many doors in life. I understood that I didn't need to starve myself to be well and slim, just to eat the right foods. This is not another silly fad diet – it is the key to being healthy.'

# The Adam & Eve Diet

*The original way to be happy, healthy and slim – for ever*

Roderick Lane and Sarah Stacey

**HODDER**

**MOBIUS**

**Please note:**
Every effort has been made by the authors to make the information in this book as clear, detailed and safe as possible. However, there may be exceptions. So we would like to point out that the procedures and concepts contained in this book are not intended as a substitute for medical advice or the advice of an appropriately trained healthcare professional.

We suggest that you undertake a basic physical examination from your doctor or appropriately qualified healthcare professional before you follow any of the programmes in this book.

If you have any health concerns of any kind, or you are pregnant or a senior citizen, you should definitely consult your doctor or an appropriately trained healthcare professional before adopting the advice given in this book.

You will see that there are places in the book (in Chapter 4 on Stress Weakness) where we counsel you to consult a doctor for advice. Please do not ignore this.

The authors and publishers do not accept any liability arising directly or indirectly from this book.

Copyright © 2002 by Roderick Lane and Sarah Stacey

First published in Great Britain in 2002 by Hodder and Stoughton
A division of Hodder Headline

The right of Roderick Lane and Sarah Stacey to be identified as the Authors of the Work has been asserted by them in accordance with the Copyright, Designs and Patents Act 1988.

10  9  8  7  6  5  4  3  2  1

A CIP catalogue record for this book is available from the British Library

ISBN 0 340 819359

Typeset by Palimpsest Book Production Limited,
Polmont, Stirlingshire
Printed and bound in Great Britain by Clays Ltd, St Ives plc

Hodder and Stoughton
A division of Hodder Headline
338 Euston Road
London NW1 3BH

# Contents

# Acknowledgements

*From Roderick Lane*

My thanks go, first and foremost, to my co-author for her patience! To our agent Kay McCauley for her unfailing support. To my colleagues Deborah Eagle and Marion Kirkham at the Naturopathic College for their insights, and to Helen Cartier-Knox and Stephanie Wright for their inspirational work and explanation for the spinal function. To each one of my patients and also Richard Day, Irene Campden and all my colleagues at Windsor who provided working examples of the different biotypes. To Paul Jayne for being my research assistant. Finally to all the teachers I have ever had for their knowledge, which laid the foundation stones for this system to be built upon.


*From Sarah Stacey*

Thanks to Rod for bringing me his knowledge, which for the first time gave me a real explanation of the way our bodies work and helped me to be fighting fit (not to speak of allowing me to eat eggs and bacon for breakfast). To Rowena Webb, Kerry Hood, Emma Heyworth-Dunn and the rest of the team at Hodder Mobius – also to our copy editor Karen Sullivan – for their extreme niceness. To Martin Welch for being a star illustrator, Lynda Brown, Leigh Richmond and Jane Phillimore for their generous help. And to Kay McCauley as ever for her endless empathy.

# How the Adam & Eve Diet Began

If you are perfectly happy with your size and shape, have boundless energy and a clear head, sleep soundly every night, never suffer from nagging illnesses and feel on top of the world most days, you probably don't need this book. If, however, you want to look and feel better, the Adam and Eve Diet can make a dramatic difference to your daily life.

You probably picked up this book because you want to lose weight – like most people in the Western world. According to recent research, nine out of 10 of us have been on a diet at some point in our lives, and this very moment half of the people around us are trying to become thinner.

Every new diet offers a new promise, and we ricochet from one to another in the vain hope of finding a regime that will solve our problems. Ultimately, we all want the same thing from food – we want to enjoy it, eat what we want when we want, feel sparkling well, both physically and mentally, and, of course, *not get fat!*

The sad truth is that the majority of diets don't work. You almost certainly won't enjoy your food, you won't feel well and, even if you do lose some weight, you are unlikely to keep it off. Research shows that most people not only put back the weight they lose, but they gain more.

The Adam and Eve Diet is different. It works.

---

## What the Adam & Eve Diet can do for you

You'll . . .

- find your perfect natural weight
- feel full of energy
- never feel hungry
- beat many chronic health problems, including insomnia, bloating, food intolerances and irritable bowel syndrome (IBS)
- enjoy your life

---

## Why does the Adam & Eve Diet work?

This revolutionary diet works because it pinpoints your individual biological type. This may sound confusing but it's quite straightforward. Your biological (bio) type is determined by the glandular biochemistry that has been handed down to you across generations, and through evolution.

There are two fundamental factors underlying this holistic approach – one is ancient, and the other is modern. First of all, medical scientists are increasingly aware that human beings are still governed by the biological traits we developed many millions of years ago, despite living in the 21st century. These are crucial to our whole make-up: physical, mental and psychological. Secondly, accompanying this legacy we have to deal with the impact of modern life – another shooting match of physical, mental and psychological pressures.

The Adam & Eve Diet was developed over many years by Roderick Lane. During his study of nutrition, he found that the concept of body typing appeared in many ancient traditional medical systems, including Ayurveda (from India) and Traditional Chinese Medicine (TCM). But far from developing a common prototype, these systems all appeared to focus on different factors, through which constitutional types were identified.

In his own clinical practice, Lane began to notice that different clients responded to different diets and to specific nutrient combinations. Clients also fell into distinct patterns, which he christened their 'Biotype'. Eventually, he identified and named five Biotypes, based on a person's dominant gland (see panel). Biotypes are confirmed when the body becomes fully formed at puberty, which is, interestingly, also the time at which we are at our physical peak. In Chapter 1, you can identify your own Biotype by answering the questionnaires.

---

### The five Biotypes

| Biotype | Dominant gland |
|---|---|
| Pathfinder | Pituitary |
| Hunter Gatherer | Thyroid |
| Pioneer | Adrenal |
| Farmer Gardener | Gonads |
| Dancer | Gonads and Pituitary |

---

Lane concluded that the five Biotypes evolved in response to the needs of early man. And those needs were all geared towards one thing: survival. Over the millennia, during which mankind evolved to its present state, there was a continuous cycle of adaptation that continues today. Just as the wily and competitive Cro Magnon pushed out the Neanderthals, another genetic mutation, the Homo sapiens, evolved between 200,000 and 100,000 years ago in response to the need to stay alive in different climates and terrains.

Lane hypothesises that the first anatomically modern Homo sapiens were 'Hunter Gatherer' types. And today's Hunter Gatherers are the descendants of the people who first walked out of prehistoric Africa to populate the world. As you will discover in Chapter 1, these Biotypes are admirably designed to roam for long distances, hunting and gathering their food as they go.

'Pathfinders', the tallest of the Biotypes, probably came next, then Pioneers, Farmer Gardeners and Dancers, the most modern in evolutionary terms. Along with their physical character-istics, these Biotypes also developed personality traits that en-abled them to adapt, and many of these are still evident today.

However, in the 21st century, we are not only the product of evolution. We are also hugely influenced by the pressures of modern living. In the Western world, we don't have to fight for enough to eat (in fact, the reverse situation exists), but if you ask people how they feel, you are unlikely to get a positive response. Sure, you'll find a few people who claim to feel very healthy and happy most of the time, but we bet that most people will say that they are anxious, tired, lacking in energy, and suffering from a chronic state of feeling one degree (and often several degrees) under par. Try it, and ask yourself, too. How do *you* feel?

Stress can place an intolerable strain on many areas of your body, including your glands (see page 13), and many of the niggling (and not so niggling) health problems experienced by the majority of the population are either caused or exacer-bated by stress.

You can identify your own individual Stress Weakness points by answering the detailed checklists in Chapter 3, and correct them by making lifestyle changes, and taking specific sup-plements, herbs and homeopathic remedies.

Because each of us is unique, it is impossible to say how long it will take to put things right, but you will begin to experience a relief of symptoms as the root problems are slowly addressed. If you've had a problem for a long time, it will take longer to correct than something less deep-seated, but the good news is that almost everything can be improved by following a few simple guidelines. If you suspect that you have a serious health condition, we advise you to consult your GP or qualified health professional immediately.

## Why the Adam & Eve Diet is revolutionary

Big claims are made for every new diet, but we believe that the Adam & Eve Diet is revolutionary. There has never, to our knowledge, been a diet that combines wisdom from both modern Western medical knowledge and traditional health care systems of the East.

The theory of this diet is simply common sense. By identifying and eating the foods that suit your specific body type, and by correcting your Stress Weaknesses, you can achieve your perfect natural weight and experience a renewed energy and zest for life.

The Biotype theory also explains a conundrum that has been foxing experts – and dieters – for decades. And this is the fact that some diets undoubtedly *do* work for some people, while they are completely ineffective for others. The explanation is that it depends on your Biotype. If you have, by chance, happened on the diet that is optimally suited to your Biotype, it will work for you (at least to some extent).

The Adam & Eve Diet takes the guesswork out of dieting. By filling in the questionnaires and identifying your Biotype and your Stress Weakness, you can pinpoint exactly the right diet for you. What's more, if you think diets are about eating nothing and feeling deprived, you'll be delighted to find that this diet is the exception. The Adam & Eve Diet is about eating deliciously, losing weight and feeling fantastic. It's certainly not about feeling hungry; in fact, the keyword is indulgence, not penance. The aim of the Adam & Eve Diet is to allow you to reach a state of optimum health and vitality – and keep you there. It works for everyone, whatever your age or state of fitness.

## The naturopathic approach

The Adam & Eve Diet is based on the naturopathic philosophy that the body will always reach towards a state of health, using its own resources to heal itself. Naturopaths believe that the body is its own best healer. They also recognise that the body, mind and spirit are interconnected and ill-health only exists when the body is not given the opportunity to self-heal.

Naturopaths describe healthcare as a three-legged stool, in which each leg is part of your life-support system. One leg represents diet, and the quality of food we eat. The second is the structure of our bodies; in particular, the spine, which is the highway between brain and body, and thus the central command system to our organs. The third leg represents the mind, spirit and psyche. It is vital to care for each leg so that the whole support system is strong and steady.

### Caring for your body

Many of us have lost the ability to listen to our bodies. We cut off at the neck and ignore messages like hunger, thirst, exhaustion, back and stomach pain, and even the need to go to the lavatory.

This book will help you to help your body, but you must be prepared to give it the attention it requires. You probably service your car regularly, and you certainly wouldn't dream of going up in an aircraft that hasn't been checked over thoroughly and refuelled. This same philosophy has to be extended to the way you care for your body. Treat it to the best grade fuel and oil, plus regular maintenance, and it will reward you with the best possible health.

### A word on cheating

Some people feel really miserable about the idea of sticking to a diet. It's fairly obvious that if you need to lose a lot of weight, you will lose it more quickly if you don't eat four bars of chocolate every day. But treats are important, too. When you start, it's essential to establish what you like to eat, and then to make sure you get it. If you just *have* to have a piece of shop-bought, full-of-additives chocolate cake or ice-cream, don't beat yourself up. Just return to your Biotype diet immediately afterwards. You will, however, find that we have provided a selection of healthy sweet treats, which should satisfy most cravings.

As your health improves, you will find that you can be more flexible. You will also find that you become more sensitive to your body's needs.

### This book can't work miracles but you can

This book is not a short-term crash diet, though there is a quick and safe weight loss plan for people who have a lot of pounds to lose. It is about living in a way that allows you to attain – and maintain – a naturally slim size and shape. As well as the optimal diet for your Biotype, with menus and basic recipes, you will find insights into your personality, plus tips on exercise, relaxation and complementary therapies.

Just one point about children: as you will read further on, the Biotypes cannot really be confirmed until after puberty. This simplifies the question of feeding a family. There is no danger – and indeed positive benefit – in children eating the same Biotype diet as their parents, since each diet is made up of a wholesome and nutritious range of freshly prepared foods.

Many hundreds of people have benefited from the Adam & Eve Diet already, and are now fighting fit. Some of their stories, including their tips and favourite recipes, are dotted throughout this book. Their lives have been transformed, and so can yours.

---

### 21 things to pick you up when you feel down (and like raiding the fridge)

Many people start a diet feeling very low. One over-weight teacher told us that she felt 'utterly miserable' about her shape and 'lack of willpower' (and those are her words, not ours).

You don't need willpower to start on this eating plan, but good will towards yourself is essential. Remember that you are worth looking after, taking time over, and feeding well. You may believe all this, but still experi-ence the odd blip when life is grey. That's when you are most vulnerable to gobbling a packet of chocolate biscuits or similar treat (the most interesting treat we heard was peanut butter sandwiches dipped in cappuccino!). You may give in to a craving when you are low, but you will undoubtedly feel worse both physically and psychologically when you do.

So, as you read through this book, keep the following advice in mind. When you feel like putting a brick through a window, or sliding into a major 'poor me' mode, try these tips for a quick, positive lift.

- Stop and breathe – slowly and rhythmically, in through your nose and out through your mouth, taking as much time to exhale as inhale.
- Make or buy a freshly squeezed juice.
- Choose a healthy snack, such as nuts and seeds.
- Dance – anywhere, everywhere – fling yourself around or just march up and down on the spot, using your arms as well as your legs.
- Give yourself a treat: buy a bunch of flowers, a magazine, bath oil or a scented candle; fix a massage or reflexology session or trade with a friend or your partner.
- Watch your favourite film on video.
- Play your favourite music: write down your own eight Desert Island Discs.
- Read your favourite novel, poem or joke.
- Listen to the radio – it's a proven fact that it lifts your mood.
- Do some gardening or have a walk in the park – getting out into nature in any shape or form will lift your spirits.
- Stroke your pets or simply go and watch animals or birds (snakes and insects, too, if you like them).
- Wear the clothes you look best in.

- Start a 'nice letters' file: put in all the letters and post-cards, invitations even, that make you feel appreciated.
- Get your sense of humour back: tell yourself a joke, look for the funny side of anything, watch a comedy on TV or video, phone an entertaining friend.
- Phone a friend who you trust, ask them to listen without interrupting and tell them the bottom line about your life, the universe and everything.
- Play the 'You're Great Game' with a friend: take a piece of paper and write down as many of the things you like about them as you can in four minutes. No 'if onlys', just 'you have lovely eyes', 'you are always sympathetic', etc. Read them aloud. Then let your friend tell you how great you are.
- Ring someone who's ill or in trouble; ask them about their problems and really listen to them.
- Make a list of what's on your mind and what you have to do, then prioritise. Give yourself one goal per day (weekends off) until you've sorted it.
- Plan an adventure – anything you like, near or far, solo or in company.
- Give yourself a hug.
- Wear your life lightly – remember that you only have today. Yesterday is gone, and tomorrow is not here. So smile, even if you fake it. Smiling and laughing send feel-good hormones scudding round your system.

# 1

## Identifying your Biotype

Your Biotype is based on your dominant gland or glands. Glands are the biochemical factories in our bodies that produce hormones, the sophisticated chemicals that regulate the whole of our body chemistry and influence all of our activities. Each gland is associated with a physiological function and this is what gives the five Biotypes their individual physical, mental and emotional characteristics.

When you are reading the descriptions of the Biotypes, remember that they are all interdependent. Each one has evolved since the time that Homo sapiens first trod the earth, and each has been altered according to their role in our global society. For this reason, there may well be overlaps, where you have one or more characteristics of another type.

Remember, too, that there are always exceptions. Because we are all individuals, there will be personal variations in body, mind and spirit. While many people fit their types exactly, others may have one feature that seems to belong to another type. For example, there can be smaller or larger versions of each type, depending on the genes you have inherited. So a man who looks like a Pathfinder because he is 6 feet 4 inches tall, but comes from a tall family and has all of the characteristics of a Hunter Gatherer, is indeed that –

a tall Hunter Gatherer. Equally, you might get a female Pioneer with the curvaceous bosom and caring nature of the Farmer Gardener. But look again, and you'll see that she lacks the hourglass torso of the Farmer Gardener and that nothing will deflect her from achieving her goals.

## The effects of stress

Your dominant gland is your strength – the roots, trunk and branches of your tree. If we had been writing this book in the early days of mankind – in fact,up until two centuries or so ago – we could have stopped here. But the last two hundred years since the Industrial Revolution have brought about huge changes to the way we live, substituting the problem of stress for the earlier and bigger question mark over survival.

Today, most of us in Western society have enough to eat and a roof over our heads. But while we do not doubt that we will survive, the majority of us live in a constant state of mental and emotional turmoil. The stress/anxiety/depression spectrum is the biggest disease state of the current age, widely recognised not only as a problem condition in its own right but also as an underlying cause behind almost every other illness, from cancer, heart disease and the degenerative diseases of ageing to colds and skin problems.

Alongside the mental and emotional stressors – including insecurities about relationships, work, money, the meaning of life and the survival of the planet – there are undoubted physical demands placed on our bodies. We live in a soup of toxic chemicals, from nicotine to petrol fumes, pesticides and herbicides to solvents in domestic and office environments, solar radiation to genetically modified ingredients in our food and even in our skincare products.

Under that toxic accumulation, even the strongest system can break down. The process of dealing with the load can put stress on our weak points, which mainly comprise the adrenal or thyroid glands, liver, blood sugar levels or spine. We call these your 'Stress Weakness Points'. In Chapter 3, you'll find comprehensive checklists to help you to identify any weakness you may have, and programmes to correct the situation.

## Stress Weakness points

Stress causes weak points in many key areas, including your glands. The glands most under pressure are the adrenals and the thyroid, and your liver and digestive system may give you problems, too. The majority of the population has back trouble at some point in their lives, and many suffer from fluctuating blood sugar levels. Whether these stress-related weaknesses are mild or severe, they can prevent you from feeling as well as you should. But once they are corrected, the transformation to both your body and mind can be startling.

The following have been identified as the main Stress Weakness points:

- Digestion
- Adrenal glands
- Thyroid gland
- Liver
- Blood sugar levels
- Spinal function

You may wonder why blood sugar irregularities are included in this section. In fact, stress has a profound effect on blood sugar, and the problem is compounded by the fact that all

13

hormones are, at one point or another, influenced by blood sugar fluctuations. For instance, when your blood sugar drops (usually because you haven't eaten), the body compensates by producing adrenaline. This raises the blood sugar level by releasing stored glucose from the liver. If blood sugar level fluctuates dramatically on a regular basis, this will affect the production of virtually all hormones.

Any of the Stress Weaknesses can affect any of the Bio-types. The symptoms don't have to be severe to affect your wellbeing; in fact, you can feel under par in a host of different ways that you cannot pinpoint, whether you are simply tired and achy, or just never feel completely healthy. The reason why we experience these problems is because the Stress Weaknesses seriously hinder the way we process and utilise food. The good news is that simple changes can often correct these weaknesses, but in some cases we recommend that you consult a qualified health professional.

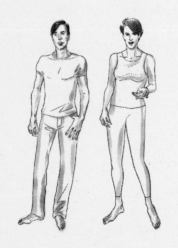

Pathfinder P
(pituitary) type

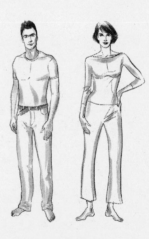

Hunter Gatherer T
(thyroid) type

As far as we know, these Stress Weaknesses have not been recognised by other nutritional experts, and identifying and addressing them can be the single most important thing you can do for your health and happiness. Alongside a diet that is appropriate for your individual Biotype, these measures will help to ensure long-lasting health and wellbeing.

## Identifying your Biotype

We've listed the five Biotypes in descending height order to make it easier for you to work out your individual type. They do not appear in order of evolution.

Pathfinder P (pituitary) type
Hunter Gatherer T (thyroid) type
Pioneer A (adrenal) type
Farmer Gardener G (gonadal) type
Dancer GP (gonadal pituitary) type

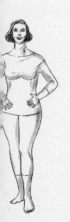

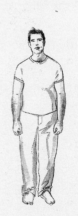

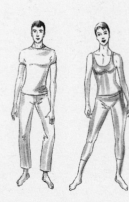

Pioneer A
(adrenal) type

Farmer Gardener G
(gonadal) type

Dancer GP
(gonadal pituitary) type

15

### Filling in the questionnaires

This is a simple process, but it is often helpful to have a friend do this with you in order to gain a true perspective of your appearance.

**Step 1**

Look at the Biotype illustrations. These represent the typical healthy shape for each Biotype. They may not be what you would consider perfect, but they are ideal – and what's more achievable. Choose the one that looks most like you. Remember there will be individual variations. Your height is a good indicator to start with, as you can see from the first illustration. If you are confused, think of the shape you are in when you look your best – often when you were in your mid-twenties.

**Step 2**

If you are overweight, look at the Fat Deposition Chart, which shows you where fat typically builds up on your Biotype. Mentally take away the excess pounds and then go to Step 3 to see which body shape you are.

Some people have no fat deposits, either because they are perfectly balanced or because they are underweight. Other people have untypical fat deposits due to events in their lives, including injuries, the use of pharmaceutical drug such as steroids, or loss of work-associated muscle structure (for instance, if a builder became a bank clerk, his unused muscles would become flabby).

If you do have fat deposits, the chart also gives you an indication of the Stress Weakness that is the likely cause of your overweight. Unless, of course, you are a doughnut addict or consistently eat a junk-food diet.

**Weight gain:** head to toe

**Stress weakness:** poor liver function

This soft, all-over fat can affect every type to some degree but is mainly found in the short Farmer Gardener types. The hourglass-become-cottage loaf look is a very good image of this type of weight gain in women, which invariably includes the dreaded dimply saddle bag weight gain on your hips and thighs. Men show all-over softness, often with some breast enlargement.

**Weight gain:** elbows to knees

**Stress weakness:** poor thyroid function

These soft deposits do not affect the face or neck, forearms or hands, calves or feet – only upper arms, torso, hips and thighs, with the most pronounced weight gain round the waist and on the abdomen and hips.

**Weight gain:** belly and bottom

**Stress weakness:** poor adrenal function

Unlike thyroid-influenced weight gain, adrenal gain is usually firm rather than dimply. The round firm 'beer gut' is a typical adrenal problem. Women put on weight fairly equally back and front, on their bottoms and stomachs.

**Step 3**

Armed with this preliminary information, complete the full Biotype questionnaire. The annotated illustrations should help you to see the most significant factors about each type. Most categories apply to both men and women; some, however, are specific to one sex. These are clearly marked.

In each category, tick the description that most closely applies to you. Think about what you look like at your optimum shape.

The Adam & Eve Diet

**Weight gain:** head to toe
**Stress weakness:** poor
liver function

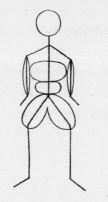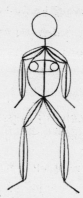

Female                                    Male

**Weight gain:** elbows to
knees
**Stress weakness:** poor
thyroid function

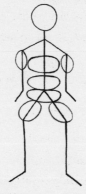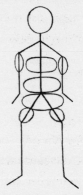

Female                                    Male

**Weight gain:** belly and
bottom
**Stress weakness:** poor
adrenal function

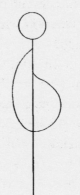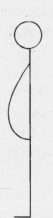

Female                                    Male

Start off by looking at yourself straight on in a full-length mirror. Later, you will need to turn sideways to inspect that view of yourself.

---

**Deceiving appearances: have you lost your waist?**

If you fit into a Biotype category except for your waist (which may seem to have disappeared) think back to when you were younger. The likelihood is that you do have a natural waist, but you have lost it because of a stress point weakness that has caused your girth to increase (see page 17).

---

1.  **Height**
    Are you:
    ☐ **A**) taller than average?
    men: over 6ft (180cm); women: over 5ft 10ins (175cm)
    ☐ **B**) average to tall?
    men: 5ft 8ins to 6 ft (170 to 180cm); women: 5ft 6ins to 5ft 10ins (165 to 175cm)
    ☐ **C**) average height?
    men: 5ft 6ins to 5ft 10ins (165 to 175cm); women: 5ft 4ins to 5ft 9ins (155 to 172.5cm)
    ☐ **D and E**) below average height?
    men: 5ft 8ins (170cm) and below; women: 5ft 4ins (155cm) and below

**2.  Hands**

Do you have:

☐ **A)** strong hands, with large and pronounced joints and knuckles?

☐ **B)** classically shaped long hands, a delicate bone structure, with fingers the same length as palms?

☐ **C)** firm hands with square, blunt fingers?

☐ **D)** soft, unbony hands with tapering but slightly full fingers?

☐ **E)** small firm hands with delicate-looking fingers?

**3.  Head and face**

Do you have:

☐ **A)** a large head, large and long face with bony nose, cheekbones and chin, etc.?

☐ **B)** a long slender face with a slight classical look?

☐ **C)** a squarish-shaped face in general, with a slight triangular cast from below the eyes to the chin?

☐ **D)** a head that appears large for your body size, with facial features that are soft, full and/or rounded as opposed to sharp?

☐ **E)** a head that seems on the small side for your body, with a neat, sharp-featured face (often described as elfin or pixie like)?

**4.  Body bone structure**

Do you have:

☐ **A)** long, strong bones with big, heavy-duty, pronounced joints?

☐ **B)** long, elegant, bird-like bones with delicate joints and wrists?

☐ **C)** short, strong, medium to heavy bones and very strong joints, supporting big muscles (particularly the biceps and calf/thigh) that are heavy fleshed?

☐ **D)** short, thick bones contrasted with joints that look delicate but are strong?

☐ **E)** short, very delicate-looking bones that are deceptively strong?

5. **Feet**

Do you have:

☐ **A)** long, narrow feet with pronounced joints and long toes, almost like fingers?

☐ **B)** longish feet with long toes and delicate bones?

☐ **C)** broad feet, well covered with flesh, toes of moderate length; feet that broaden toward the toes although heels may be narrow?

☐ **D)** small, soft feet, often described as baby- or child-like, with short stubby toes; feet are even shaped and non-tapering, with heels almost as wide as toes?

☐ **E)** as above, but with feet that taper towards the heel?

6. **Chest and torso**

*Women*

Do you have:

☐ **A)** a strong rib cage with large collar bones and medium to large breasts

☐ **B)** a long, quite delicate-looking rib cage, which is usually very narrow seen from the side, with small to medium-sized breasts?

☐ **C)** a large ribcage and torso, which is thick and big seen from the side, with medium to large breasts; torso often looks as though you have spent a lot of time in sports training, such as swimming or athletics?

☐ **D**) a full, soft-looking rib cage with medium to large breasts?

☐ **E**) a small, delicate-looking rib cage, almost like a teenager, with medium to small breasts

*Men*

Do you have:

☐ **A**) a strong rib cage with large collar bones?

☐ **B**) a long, narrow, more delicate-looking rib cage?

☐ **C**) a large rib cage and torso, which is big viewed from the side with an obvious underlying muscle structure, as though you have played contact sports or lifted weights?

☐ **D**) a rather barrel-chested, soft-looking rib cage with poorly defined muscle structure?

☐ **E**) a small, light-boned rib cage, almost adolescent in structure?

Now turn so that you can see your side view.

**7.   General build**

Do you see:

☐ **A**) a long body, flattish rather than curvy and/or contoured, with long legs and strong joints, on an overall large scale?

☐ **B**) an overall long and lean tendency, with a long fine torso balanced by longish, well-shaped legs; a bone structure that tends to be refined and delicate?

☐ **C**) a strong torso with compact muscular legs and a prominent rear balanced by a prominent chest?

☐ **D**) a short figure in general, with short legs in proportion to the rest of the body, poorly defined muscles, a prominent rear and chest, with pronounced waist and hips in women?

☐ E) a relatively straight flat torso, with a very adolescent look to it; body structure tends to look delicate or even weak but is actually very strong with whip cord muscle?

8. **Upper and lower body**

Now compare your upper body to your lower body, ignoring body fat.

*Women*

Do you see:

☐ A) a straight-sided torso with very little definition at the waist, which goes into only slightly more prominent hips?

☐ B) a torso that tapers slightly to a moderately pronounced waist, with fairly prominent hips and thighs?

☐ C) a torso that is wide at the top, tapering down only slightly to the waist, with strong legs and thighs, and hips approximately the same width as upper torso?

☐ D) an hourglass figure with full bosom, curvy hips and a wasp waist; body may be covered with a soft watery layer of fat?

☐ E) a delicate-looking torso and ribs, shoulders the same width as hips, and a barely defined waist; body tends to look physically young, almost teenage, even if the face shows signs of ageing.

*Men*

Do you see:

☐ A) a torso that goes straight down at the sides with very little waist definition; underlying big bone structure is clearly visible?

☐ **B)** a torso that slightly tapers to the waist; a naturally slender abdomen with poorly defined muscle structure?

☐ **C)** a wide-shouldered torso that tapers down to the waist, very chunky abdomen and strong legs and thighs, with hips approximately the same width as the upper torso?

☐ **D)** a rounded chest contrasting with straight-sided body, overlaid by a soft layer of body fat?

☐ **E)** shoulders in line with hips, slight waist, slight-looking torso and ribs; body tends to look physically young, almost teenage, even if face shows signs of ageing?

### Scoring

If you score 6 or more in one category (A, B, C, D or E), you fall into the corresponding Biotype.

> **A** = Pathfinder
> **B** = Hunter Gatherer
> **C** = Pioneer
> **D** = Farmer Gardener
> **E** = Dancer

In Chapter 2, you'll find the diet guidelines for your particular Biotype, with menus, recipes, store-cupboard tips and a directory later in the book.

### What to do if you can't identify your Biotype

If you score 5 or under, you should turn to Chapter 3 and fill in the Stress Weakness checklists because your physical type has almost certainly been affected by a stress-induced condition. The most common physical result is weight gain, as we have explained earlier in this chapter (see page 16). The probable causes of Stress Weaknesses are listed below.

As you follow the Stress Weakness programme for your

most significant problem, your body will start to achieve a state of balance. As this happens, your energy level will change and your body shape will begin to return to its natural Biotype. After four weeks, go back to Step 3 of the Biotype questionnaire and fill it in again. If you don't get a clear outcome, repeat on a monthly basis until you do.

Stressful life experiences that may affect your physical type:

- You were born prematurely – premature babies often fail to develop to their full natural potential; for instance, their hands or feet remain small.
- You have been consistently overweight for most of your life.
- You have been a consistent dieter throughout your life.
- You have been seriously ill or suffered a chronic health problem that has caused weight loss.
- You have, at some point, spent a considerable amount of time doing weight training, following a comprehensive exercise programme or training for another activity that has affected the way you grow. Swimming, rugby, football, weight-lifting and training, for example, all place stress on the muscular skeletal system and muscular overdevelopment can alter your shape. There are other, rarer causes of muscular overdevelopment; for example, flute players' fingers may grow longer as a result of trying to reach all the notes.
- You have been on a pharmaceutical or other drug that has induced a change in your body shape, and the level and/or distribution of body fat. Drugs that may do this include: steroids and hormones which alter the growth pattern and development of muscles; chemotherapy or radiation therapy, which do the same thing and may also cause loss

of muscle mass; or hard drugs, which can change body muscle density. In this case, you should move on to the Stress Weakness checklists in Chapter 3.

## Biotype characteristics

### Biotype 1 *Pathfinder*
### Gland     *Pituitary*

**Famous Pathfinders**

| | |
|---|---|
| Jerry Hall | Uma Thurman |
| Venus Williams | Christina Dodwell |
| Cameron Diaz | |

| | |
|---|---|
| Ranulf Fiennes | Jeremy Paxman |
| Jeremy Vine | Liam Neeson |
| Bill Clinton | Duke of Edinburgh |
| Vinny Jones | Tom Hanks |
| Laurence Fishburne | |

Pathfinders are the trail-blazers – hardy, self-contained and independent. They are scouts, striking out across new territories, often on their own. Explorer Christina Dodwell, who travels solo, is a typical example of a modern woman Pathfinder. As a type, the tall rangy Pathfinder probably evolved after the Hunter Gatherers, to protect the needs of their communities when crises such as famine struck, and the group needed to move on. The inquisitive but dreamy Hunter Gatherers are more likely to have adventured to a new terrain before the need became pressing. But when the time came to explore it properly, the more practical Pathfinders would come along and hack back the trail for the Pioneers and Farmer Gardeners. The Pathfinder is the one we look to now

Height:
over 6ft
(180cm)

Height:
over 5ft
10ins
(175cm)

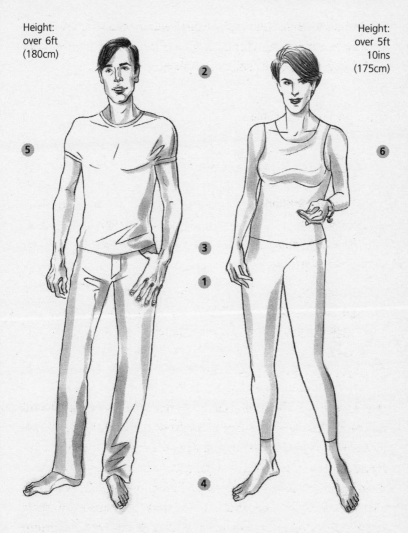

**The Pathfinder** A long body, flattish rather than curvy or contoured, with long legs and strong joints.

**1** Strong hands, with large and pronounced joints and knuckles.

**2** A large head, large and long face, with bony nose, cheekbones and chin.

**3** Long, strong bones with heavy-duty, pronounced joints.

**4** Long, narrow feet with pronounced joints and long toes, almost like fingers.

**5** *Men*: a strong ribcage with large collarbones.

**6** *Women*: a strong ribcage with large collarbones and medium to large breasts.

when a state of radical change has to be initiated – the Hunter Gatherer will dream it up, the Pathfinder and the Pioneer will make it happen.

**Physical type**

The pituitary gland is associated with growth hormones and thus the growth of bones, joints and muscles. Look at the drawings of the Pathfinder man and woman and you will see their large build, brought about by pituitary gland dominance. They have the heaviest bones and all of the bony areas – forehead, nose, chin, chest, knees, etc. – are big. Long hands with big bony knuckles are always a giveaway. Due to their physical size, however, they can look thin, even emaciated. Pathfinders are prone to arthritic conditions, mainly because of their tendency to ignore aches and pains. Their attitude is to forget their problems in the hope that they'll go away.

Because the pituitary gland and gonads function at opposite ends of the metabolic seesaw, Pathfinder women often have low oestrogen and/or progesterone, and a tendency to pre-menstrual syndrome (PMS). When they are well, Pathfinders have incredible reserves of energy and are up with the larks, getting on with the day.

**Mental and emotional tendencies**

'Mustn't grumble' is one of the most likely things you'll hear from a Pathfinder man or woman. Laid-back and more or less unflappable, they are the ultimate stoics. Confront them with a problem and they will just get on and deal with it. They will give up smoking, drinking, drug-taking and lovers overnight and grit their teeth as they go through cold turkey.

They are often kind but may sometimes be seen as uncaring

because they often fail to respond overtly to other people's emotional needs. Due to an innate determination to be physically indestructible, they tend to ignore physical problems and find it hard to understand them in others. This type of approach is typical:

Pathfinder to absent employee: 'You mean you're not coming in because you think you've got flu? I was in last week with a broken leg and my wife/husband/child was in hospital.'

You might well find the Pathfinder in your life mending your car, partly because they're concerned about your safety but also because they can't face the irritation of you being late to meet them. Pathfinders are the dark horse Biotype: they observe everything but may never reveal it. If they're interested in a subject or a person, however, they will make themselves masters of detail. They make great captains of industry, explorers and leaders of any kind – look at the Duke of Wellington and the explorer Christina Dodwell. Because they tend not to recognise limits of any kind, they may also be visionary in their approach to almost any area in their lives, from career to romance. They tend to have a black-and-white view of life: they are right and, yes, you are wrong. So they also do well as barristers or accountants.

**Biotype 2 *Hunter Gatherer***
**Gland      *Thyroid***

**Famous Hunter Gatherers**

| | |
|---|---|
| Darcey Bussell | Rene Russo |
| Iman | Halle Berry |
| Diana, Princess of Wales | Elizabeth Hurley |

Joseph Fiennes          Terence Stamp
Robert Carlyle          Richard Branson
Johnny Depp

As we explained earlier, the first three people who walked out of the cradle of Africa and populated the rest of the world were probably Hunter Gatherers. In the Hunter Gatherer we find man's first curious being and the first evolutionary type – people who are the most in tune with nature's rhythms. For them, the act of movement is instinctive and part of their basic survival strategy. They are nomadic, fretful if asked to sit still because they are designed to walk long distances, gathering food as they go.

At times of crisis, when a group of people needed to move on because the grazing was depleted or the soil exhausted (or the modern equivalent, for instance, new ways of farming or doing business), the Hunter Gatherers were in their element. They had been over the mountain, or exploring that far off green valley, simply because they wanted to see what was there.

Today, Hunter Gatherers are often happiest dreaming up new schemes, ambitious as you like, then working in tandem with the Pathfinders and their second-in-commands, the Pioneers, to make them happen, before the Farmer Gardeners settle in for the longer term.

### Physical type

The thyroid gland produces the hormone thyroxin, which sets the metabolic rate, also called the rate of energy conversion. This is the rate at which we burn stored energy. Hunter Gatherers tend to have a slow pulse and low blood pressure and can keep going almost indefinitely. They are built for

Height:
5ft 8ins to 6ft
(170cm
to180cm)

Height:
5ft 6ins to
5ft 10ins
(165cm to
175cm)

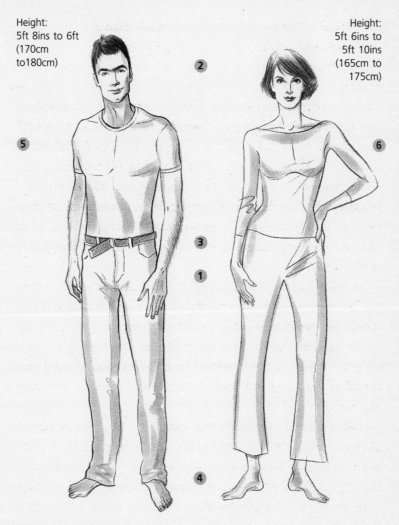

**The Hunter Gatherer** An overall long and lean tendency, with a long torso balanced by longish well-shaped legs.

**1** Classically shaped long hands, a delicate bone structure, with fingers the same length as palms.

**2** A long, slender face with a slightly classical look.

**3** Long, elegant, bird-like bones with delicate joints and wrists.

**4** Longish feet with long toes and delicate bones.

**5** *Men*: a long, narrow, delicate-looking ribcage.

**6** *Women*: a long, quite delicate-looking ribcage, narrow from the side, with small to medium breasts.

31

endurance, walking, jogging, hunting and gathering, but not weight-lifting.

They will walk for hours with long loping strides and a graceful gliding gait. Their stamina is virtually limitless as long as they keep at a moderate consistent rate; make them run however and they will (literally) run out of energy very quickly.

Hunter Gatherers tend to suffer from chronic nagging problems such as neck or shoulder ache, blocked sinuses and skin rashes. Physically they tend to be reserved: quiet rather than boisterous, gentle rather than grabbing at people or things. Grasp a Hunter Gatherer's hand too strongly and they will recoil.

Female Hunter Gatherers often make supermodels. Often one of their most notable features is a long swan-like neck. They tend to have fine, dry skin, which may age into lines and wrinkles if they don't have enough essential fatty acids (EFAs) in their diet, including oily fish and supplements such as oil of evening primrose and flaxseed.

**Mental and emotional tendencies**

Women Hunter Gatherers are usually very graceful and the men have a well-developed sensitive side. They tend to be dreamers and romantics so they are often very creative. They love travelling, whether it's misty morning walks through the park or jetting off to Colorado to ride down the Rockies. Highly sensual in every way, they are also very artistic, so their environment and also their work is likely to be imaginative, inventive and attractive. Colours, shapes, textures and sounds are very important to them.

Unlike Pathfinders, Hunter Gatherers see things as shades of grey, rather than black and white. They are thoughtful, tending to need time to consider problems rather than giving an immediate answer. They will often negotiate and compromise. These traits may make them seen – incorrectly – as ineffectual or weak by some.

They can be like terriers with issues, refusing to let go until they have gently but fully explained the significance. They may find it hard to accept (and even hear!) their listener saying 'yes' and can start rehashing an argument even when the other has agreed to their points. Because they are very moral and mystical, they find it hard to understand that others will agree to something they don't fully believe, in order to have a quiet life.

Hunter Gatherers gather. They tend to have all sorts of collections around them, from overflowing bowls of fruit and baskets of vegetables, to pebbles, feathers, stamps, paper clips, bits of ribbon and string, computer programmes, CDs, lofts full of suitcases, old photos and so on. You name it, they gather it. They may also gather people as causes and as friends. In fact, they are usually charming and sociable and empathetic. Their mystical side means that they are often effective healers, although they have to be careful not to become exhausted.

They can appear contradictory when it comes to displays of affection: sometimes demonstrative physically, loving to hug and cuddle, other times reticent and chilly. It just depends on who they are with.

Hunter Gatherers tend to work things out in their heads, which is great for mental arithmetic and debating, but often not so good for relationships. They tend to rehash events and conversations in an internal dialogue which, necessarily, doesn't include the other person/s. This means, of course, that they may reach inaccurate conclusions. The upside is that they can be marvellous listeners and are usually clamlike when asked to keep a secret.

Careerwise, they tend to gravitate to the arts – which satisfies their creative side – mathematics or music. They enjoy precision, and professions that use their ability to empathise and communicate.

### Biotype 3 *Pioneer*
### Gland      *Adrenal*

**Famous Pioneers**

| | |
|---|---|
| Catherine Zeta-Jones | Angelina Jolie |
| Meg Ryan | Susan Sarandon |
| Anne Bancroft | Tea Leoni |
| | |
| Richard Gere | Russell Crowe |
| Antonio Banderas | Bruce Willis |
| Mark Baldwin | Michael Flatley |

Pioneer types are one of the most numerous Biotypes. This stalwart and determined adaptation evolved through the necessity, over many generations, of enabling men and women to push themselves through difficult situations. They have an incredible will to get things done, and never give up. 'Onward and upward' could be the Pioneer's mantra.

The Pioneer comes to the fore when the community needs to move on, with all its goods, chattels and herds. The physical strength and single-mindedness of the Pioneer enables them to carry the burden of their family on their back – sometimes literally.

The Pioneer is the person you want around when it's a question of survival, or of achieving a deadline. They're in

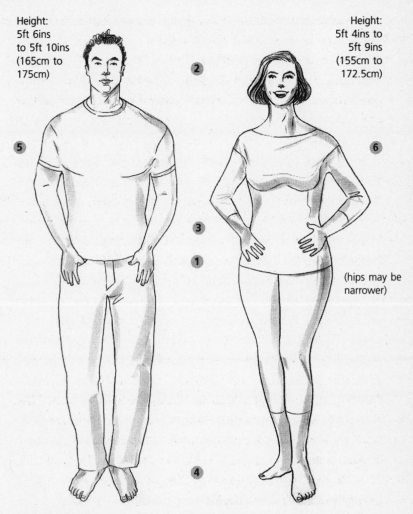

Height:
5ft 6ins
to 5ft 10ins
(165cm to
175cm)

Height:
5ft 4ins to
5ft 9ins
(155cm to
172.5cm)

(hips may be
narrower)

**The Pioneer** A strong torso with compact muscular legs and a prominent rear balanced by a prominent chest.

**1** Firm hands with square, blunt fingers.

**2** A squarish face with a slight triangular cast from below the eyes to the chin.

**3** Short, strong, medium to heavy bones and very strong joints supporting big muscles, particularly biceps, thighs and calves.

**4** Broad feet, well covered with flesh, toes of moderate length and feet that broaden towards the toes.

**5** *Men*: a large ribcage and torso, with an obvious underlying muscle structure.

**6** *Women*: a large ribcage and torso, which is thick and big; medium to large breasts.

35

their element then, never stopping, never questioning, just getting on with it. They won't expect to be thanked either. If you want your spirits lifting, call a Pioneer. They'll help you sort your problems, organise a party *and* tell you jokes along the way.

**Physical type**

The adrenal glands produce adrenaline, the fight or flight hormone that enabled early man to battle the mountain lion, sabre toothed tiger or rival tribes. Pioneer types are capable of incredible bursts of concentration and energy, and have the ability to push on through emergency situations. Think of the pioneer men and women rolling their wagon trains through the American West. They tend to be sprinters, running round at top speed then suddenly coming to a full stop. Pioneers are the ones who fall asleep in their soup at dinner. Their energy supplies can shut down as instantly as they fire up. Pioneers tend to suffer from impact injuries such as damaged knees or backs; they are also the classic sufferers of stress-related illnesses which, due to their innate impatience, are never allowed to repair fully. They can be prone to heart problems, and have to take extra care because they may also have addictive personalities.

**Mental and emotional tendencies**

Pioneers are the salt of the earth. They tend to like working – and playing – in teams (think of the wagon trains) in a situation where structure is imposed on them in some way. Male Pioneers tend to be the ultimate in masculinity, strong, fearless, dependable and self-sufficient. Although these blokey blokes generally like and appreciate women, they may have difficulty connecting and communicating with them emotionally.

Women Pioneers, like Farmer Gardener women, tend to be good organisers and 'jolly hockeysticks' types: the ones who carried on driving the wagon trains out West when their menfolk were dead and the arrows whistled round them. These days they organise anything from fêtes and charity balls to children's sports days and conferences. Pioneers are goal-orientated, carrying on through every obstacle until the job is done. However, the need to push on can blind them to the best decision, so they're often not the best choice for leader. In most cases, they make better second in commands and can be phenomenal organisers and motivators if well directed.

Firm and true, once a Pioneer has said they're your friend, you have them for life. The downside for other types, such as the romantic Hunter Gatherers, is that they may never tell you twice. ('I told you I loved you 20 years ago, so you must know it.') Note, too, that these opposites – the Hunter Gatherer and the Pioneer – often attract!

Their food preferences tend to be simple and their hobbies physical. Unlike the sensual Hunter Gatherers, Pioneers could easily live in a hotel room and their houses quite often look like that – spick and span, neat as a new pin, with little identity and few messy knickknacks. Conversely, they may totally ignore where they live since it's just where they return to sleep, shower and change. In this case, home is likely to resemble a tip.

But don't let the Pioneers' practical upper side lead you to think that they don't have a romantic and creative soul – it just needs to be uncovered.

**Biotype 4 *Farmer Gardener***
**Gland      *Gonads***

**Famous Farmer Gardeners**

| | |
|---|---|
| Ivana Trump | Drew Barrymore |
| Sophia Loren | Gillian Anderson |
| Dolly Parton | Sarah Michelle Geller |
| Barbara Windsor | |
| | |
| Sir Anthony Hopkins | Robin Williams |
| Mel Gibson | Bob Hoskins |

Although they are usually energetic and full-of-life characters, Farmer Gardeners represent the more static nature of man. Once a community reaches new pastures, it needs feeding, and that's where Farmer Gardeners come into their own. They are designed to nurture: to plant seeds, raise livestock and produce children. Today the caring professions are filled with this Biotype. And they do it remarkably well, shouldering responsibility willingly and uncomplainingly. Civilisations are built on the stability of Farmer Gardeners.

**Physical type**
The gonadal glands produce the reproductive hormones, testosterone, oestrogen and progesterone. Farmer Gardener Biotypes, who are characterised by round, soft body fat and prominent sexual features, look fertile and nurturing, particularly the hourglass-shaped women. Men tend to have hair sprouting all over: chest and neck, back, arms and wrists. If they put on weight, they tend to do a cross between a waddle and a strut.

Farmer Gardeners often have a history of eating poorly with related weight gain; because of this they are also prone

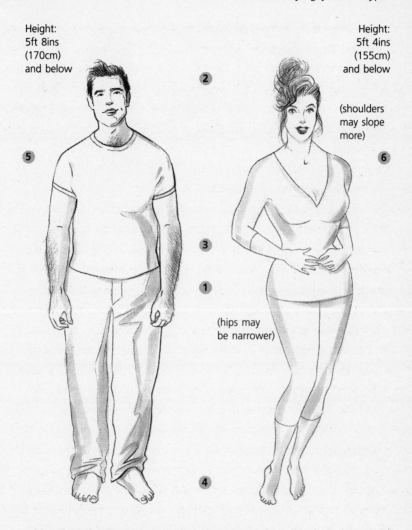

Height:
5ft 8ins
(170cm)
and below

Height:
5ft 4ins
(155cm)
and below

(shoulders
may slope
more)

(hips may
be narrower)

**The Farmer Gardener** A short figure, with short legs (in proportion), prominent rear and chest, and pronounced waist and hips in women.
**1** Soft, unbony hands with tapered but slightly full fingers.
**2** A large head, soft and full rounded facial features.
**3** Short, thick bones and delicate but strong joints.
**4** Small, soft feet with short, stubby toes; non-tapering from heels to toes.
**5** *Men*: a barrel-chested, soft-looking ribcage, with poorly defined musculature.
**6** *Women*: a full, soft-looking ribcage, with medium to large breasts.

39

to bad backs and knees. And because of their hormonally dominated make-up, women Farmer Gardeners are prone to PMS.

Farmer Gardeners can change their shape by exercising to extremes – they take on the look of their semi-counterpart the Dancer – but the problem is that as soon as they stop, they run to seed.

## Mental and emotional tendencies

Farmer Gardeners tend to have a high libido and caring natures. They are the quintessential nurturers, following professions such as doctor, nurse, teacher, social worker, office manager, cook, full-time parent and, of course, farmer and gardener. They're the ones who will make sure that the children/grandparents/livestock/workers are fed and watered, and tucked up properly at night.

Farmer Gardeners usually have tremendous enthusiasms. They are often in love with being in love so they have crushes and fall in love passionately. They are ferociously protective of their families: threaten their children and they turn into tigers or tigresses immediately. Farmer Gardeners are loyal and reliable, hard-working and self-sacrificing, but they may hold a grudge for eternity.

Farmer Gardeners tend to undervalue their own worth, so they work hard and conscientiously, seldom giving themselves a break. This Biotype will work late every night, be back first in the office after flu, and offer to shoulder other peoples' loads. Such dedication can result in stress-related conditions.

Farmer Gardeners can be very good at listening to other people and considerate of their needs – although that may be partnered by gossiping about them, too. Seldom martyrs, their positive personality shines through even the most difficult circumstances and they can throw themselves into having fun – often proving the life and soul of the party.

Farmer Gardeners are quintessentially homemakers. Their energy is concentrated in the environment in which they and their family live. They are also often image conscious and, because they like to collect things, will have collections of knickknacks – anything from china and paintings to boxes and their favourite collectable. Jewellery tends to be a collectable for both sexes.

They are offerers of hospitality. This is the Biotype that can be depended on to welcome you with a cup of tea, home-made goodies, a seat by the fire (or its equivalent) and a nice chat. Their fridge will be full and the store cupboard stuffed with emergency rations. What's more, if you've grazed your hand, they will know where the packet of plasters is and have made certain that it isn't empty. But don't expect soppy treatment: they are wonderful carers and nurses but they expect obedience, so no messing about.

This Biotype is the linchpin of the family, keeping in touch with parents and children alike, even distant cousins. They have a social conscience that shines in their own community rather than on a larger scale – popping round to see a sick neighbour rather than fretting too much about far-flung problems.

## Biotype 5 *Dancer*
**Glands** *Pituitary and Gonads*

**Famous Dancers**

| | |
|---|---|
| Winona Ryder | Ann Robinson |
| Christina Ricci | Lucy Liu |
| Deborah Bull | |

Tom  Cruise          Michael J. Fox
Jasper  Conran

Dancers are the most recent type to emerge – some 30 or 40,000 years ago . . . They are the product of two Biotypes – the Pathfinder and the Farmer Gardener – gravitating together. You can still see these two Biotypes walking along the street today: a towering  footballer or rower, for instance, hand in hand with a diminutive Dolly Parton-type who hardly comes up to his chest. Clinical experience suggests that they may well produce Dancer children, although not invariably.

The difference between Dancers and the other Biotypes is that the first four (Pathfinder, Hunter Gatherer, Pioneer and Farmer Gardener) were all survival adaptations brought about by the exigencies of living in the wild, with tigers on their tail or another ice age round the corner. Dancers, however, are the ultimate urban people. They developed because of a changing social culture, when the world population started to live more structured and stable lives, creating villages, cities, kingdoms and, later, empires.

Charming and determined, with a wacky sense of humour, Dancers combine both the dynamic nature of the Pathfinder, needed to survive in large crowds, and the stability of the Farmer Gardener. They are eminently adaptable and flexible and can respond very quickly to changing social and environmental conditions.

Mankind is still evolving worldwide and, over the next decades and centuries, we expect a lessening of the original survival types and more combinations.

Height:
5ft 8ins
(170cm)
and below

Height:
5ft 4ins
(155cm)
and below

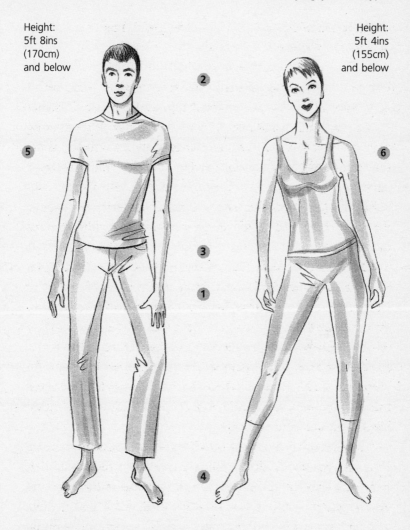

**The Dancer** A straight, flat torso, with a delicate, adolescent body structure that is very strong.
**1** Small, firm hands with delicate-looking fingers.
**2** A small head with a neat, sharp-featured face.
**3** Short, delicate-looking bones that are deceptively strong.
**4** Small, soft feet that taper towards the heel.
**5** *Men*: a small, light-boned ribcage, almost adolescent.
**6** *Women*: a small, delicate-looking ribcage with medium to small breasts.

43

**Physical type**

The Dancer Biotype is the only one to combine two dominant glands and thus two hormonal functions, pituitary (like
the Pathfinder) and gonadal (like the Farmer Gardener). In
the case of the Dancer, however, the pituitary gland provides
not growth (Dancers are the shortest of the Biotypes) but
strength of bone and ligament. The gonads provide the sexual
hormones that give Dancers their trademark delicate appearance. This belies their physical strength: Dancers are iron
butterflies. Ballet dancers, for instance, are a perfect example:
they look ethereal as they waft around on stage but are as
physically tough as bantam weight boxers. They can take
incredible physical punishment, but they will suffer as a result.
They are prone to damaged joints and aching muscles with
chronic problems such as neck- or backache.

**Mental and emotional tendencies**

Small and fiery, Dancers are often highly amusing and entertaining – and very quick-witted. Careerwise, they are versa-
tile. They often work well in the arts or in other creative
professions where strength, dedication and discipline are
needed in equal measure. Their drive will take them to the
top, but then they may suddenly upsticks and move on to
another. Dancers tend to get swept up in the mood of the
moment, rising to any occasion, and then exit when it suits
them. They tend to be erratic emotionally, too, swinging
from sensitive and loving to unconcerned, even offhand, in
a flash.

Dancers are contradictory in some ways, partly due to their
combination of glandular types. They have an iron will and,
impelled by their Pathfinder pituitary dominance, they think
they can cope with anything. But they may get in over their

heads and their Farmer Gardener gonads may not be able to cope under extreme pressure.

Their weak spot is that they tend to have addictive personalities that can manifest in different ways, from addictive behaviour – in almost any area you can think of, from shopping to work, to romance and sex – to full-blown addictions, such as alcoholism, drug addiction or eating disorders. They will be wholeheartedly extreme about something or someone, learn everything about it or them, then suddenly drop the subject like a hot potato and go off in a completely different direction.

Dancers' lives may seem like firing ranges, but they also crave tranquillity. Emotionally, they tend to be cool, holding everything inside – until they explode. Dancers are real 'sh*t hits the fan' people at that point. Their communication skills are good, but they find it hard to negotiate with people who don't see their point of view.

A typical Dancer statement in a difficult situation might be: 'I've told him/her but they still don't understand; it is pointless even trying to talk to them about that.'

Dancers tend to like simplicity, just as long as it's sophisticated – like them. Go into a Dancer's house and you will likely find Shaker furniture and Philippe Starck details, or sleek equivalents. Looks wise, they are self-aware and very conscious of their own image. They tend to like being in the forefront of fashion, following the latest trends, though not originating them (that's more likely to be a dreamy, creative Hunter Gatherer).

Just like the ballet dancers they are named after, Dancer Biotypes are light on their toes, both physically and mentally – mercurial people who can see the humour in every situation and believe that every cloud has a silver lining.

# 2

## The Biotype Diets

The Adam & Eve Diet is successful because it is simple. As we discussed earlier, different Biotypes have adapted through evolution, and each of these types thrives on different ways of eating. And that, in a nutshell, is the principle of this diet.

Because there is only a handful of food groups – meats, fish, vegetables/salad/fruits, grains, nuts and seeds – and because we all tend to have more or less the same patterns of eating times, the differences may seem small. Don't be misled. Subtle shifts can bring radical results.

Before we start on the specifics of each eating plan, there are some general guidelines to remember. First of all, let's focus on treats! It's very important that you know you can have a treat every day. You may not want one, but if you do, it's completely acceptable. Secondly, although the advice on shopping and cooking is not cast in stone, the closer you stay to the programme, the better you will feel and the more quickly the changes will take place.

### Treat yourself

**Alcohol:** You will see that alcohol comes into the 'Try To Avoid' category, but if you crave alcohol, do allow yourself a couple of glasses of good wine a day – mixed with fizzy water or soda as a spritzer, if you wish.

**Coffee:** If you love coffee, allow yourself one or two cups of freshly made, organic (that's important) coffee daily, preferably in the morning so that you don't risk sleeping poorly. It's best if you can drink decaffeinated, but don't drive yourself mad over it. If you can't get organic decaffeinated (and you really should try), choose brands that are water washed (in other words, the caffeine is removed by water, not ethanol). All organically produced, decaffeinated teas and coffees are water washed, which means that you are taking in fewer chemicals.

**Chocolate:** If you crave the taste of chocolate during the first 14 days of your Biotype diet, go for a carob sweetmeat from the healthfood shop. After that, reward yourself with a square or two of organic chocolate daily, if you wish. Let it melt on your tongue for maximum taste sensation. There are some healthy sweet treats listed on on page 54 and in the recipe section – a delicious and satisfying alternative.

**Days off:** Allow yourself one or two half days off your diet every fortnight. Eat your normal breakfast and lunch, then eat and drink whatever you want for the rest of the day.

Other points to remember:

- Wherever possible, eat fresh, unprocessed and organic foods (see below). This includes meat and dairy produce. We do not mention organic food specifically in the diets below, but we suggest that you will choose organic brands wherever possible, over their non-organic counterparts. Organic food is superior in every way to non-organic, and can make a big difference to your overall health.
- Potatoes are a relatively 'new' root vegetable, and should be eaten sparingly by all types. They do not, for this reason,

fall into the category of 'root vegetables', unless specifically mentioned.

- Eat foods that are in season.
- Try to avoid all conventionally reared pork and pork products (such as pies, ham and bacon) because they tend to carry even more additives than other conventionally reared livestock; pork also has a high fat content. The occasional organic bacon or ham treat is fine, however.
- Avoid tinned (canned) or packaged produce. It usually has less nutritional value and often contains added sugar and salt. Some tinned fish (in particular, deep-sea fish such as tuna and sardines) is acceptable, however, because it is frozen and canned immediately and is, therefore, relatively free of additives and pollutants.
- If you can't find fresh fruit or vegetables, frozen are fine and there is now an extensive range of organic frozen produce.
- Many people are intolerant to modern wheat products. Look for primitive grains, such as spelt, faro, kamut and quinoa (see page 55), now widely available at healthfood stores and good supermarkets. These are less likely to trigger allergic or intolerance reactions.
- Use organic, cold pressed, extra virgin oil in food preparation and cooking. Grill or cook in a wok. Avoid deep- or shallow-frying: it can raise the calorie content of some foods by 1500 per cent, and is a powerful source of free radicals (which are implicated in serious cell damage that can lead to conditions such as cancer and heart disease).
- Remember that conventionally grown coffee and tea are treated with larger amounts of non-organic fertilisers, herbicides and pesticides than any other crops – so choose organically produced brands wherever possible.

- Check that flavoured teas or drinks do not contain synthetic flavourings or additives.
- All types do well on freshly juiced organic vegetables and fruit; see Chapter 6 for suggested combinations and a good detox regime. In fact, all types should include a fresh juice at breakfast or as a pick-me-up during the day.

### Why choose organic food?

Naturopaths believe that good food is the foundation of life and health and that the quality of the foods we eat is reflected in our lives. Nourish your body with the best possible food and it will reward you with gleaming health.

Fresh, unprocessed food is always best, but organically produced food is best of all. We recommend organic food not so much for its improved nutrient content, but because it contains far fewer (and in most cases no) artificial chemicals.

We live our daily lives in a soup of chemicals from many different sources. Singly, they may not harm us, but put them all together and it can amount to a chemical assault and battery. Where we have the choice – as we do in the case of food – it makes sense to opt for the most healthy option. It is not an efficient use of our bodies' energy to expend part of the nutrients we absorb from food in purging ourselves of synthetic chemicals from that same food. Take your average apple, for example. It may have been sprayed up to 50 times with pesticides before reaching the supermarket shelves, and probably languished in the back of a lorry for some time before it was ready for sale. It may have been treated with waxes and other chemicals to maintain its appearance and lengthen its shelf life. The vitamins and minerals found in that apple will likely have declined to almost nothing by the time we come to eat it, and what little nutrition there is will be required by our bodies to detoxify the chemicals that were used to treat it. In reality, therefore, that apple gives us nothing at all.

When we eat conventionally produced foods – both plant crops and meat, poultry and fish – we run the risk of consuming a cocktail of chemicals that we never agreed to take. While individual chemicals are tested and declared 'safe', cocktails of these same chemicals have never been tested and they are more than capable of having unknown and long-term effects in our bodies. Plant crops may contain the residues of fertilisers, pesticides and herbicides. Intensively reared livestock are routinely given drugs to ward off illness and to increase their output and weight. This includes antibiotics in cattle, which are used both to prevent illness and to promote growth, and antimicrobial drugs in poultry for the table. Non-organic eggs (even free range) may also contain chemical residues. We are particularly concerned about pork and pork products because pigs have a high fat content, which provides a perfect storage place for all forms of toxins that may then be passed on to the consumer.

There are further obvious causes for concern over 'factory farmed' animals that may be fed on the ground-up remains of other animals. Many naturally vegetarian animals, for example, are forced onto a high protein carnivorous diet. BSE came about for precisely this reason. The disease then, as we know, passed the species barrier and has already caused the deaths of 99 people at the time of writing this book.

Organic farming aims to avoid the use of artificial chemical fertilisers and pesticides on the land, relying instead on developing a healthy fertile soil and growing a mixture of crops. Organically reared animals are not routinely treated with prophylactic drugs and disease of any kind is often treated with homeopathy and herbs (even acupuncture and chiropractic). What's more, no organic food can contain artificial ingredients that do not conform to rigid organic standards, set by certification bodies and stringently upheld. When you choose organic, you know you are getting something that is as free from toxins as any modern food can be.

## Ad speak – not!

Much of our diet today is dictated by advertisements and poor dietary advice. Before you get started on the Adam & Eve Diet, it's important to know the key facts about the food we eat, and the reason why we need to make changes.

### Buttering us up

The advertisements tell us that we should give up butter and use margarine because it's good for lowering cholesterol. In fact, margarine is a manmade product containing hydrogenated fat, which is difficult for the system to break down and utilise properly. What's more, it is a source of dangerous 'transfatty' acids, which are linked to many health problems, including cancer.

Butter, however, is a natural product that contains vitamins, enzymes, fats and minerals needed for good health. Choose it instead, whenever possible, and buy organic to make an even greater difference. We should note here that some of the newer margarines on the market are not conventionally produced, and therefore bring the many health benefits of pure, good-quality vegetable oils. We list these, for your convenience, in the Store-cupboard recommendations (see page 269).

### White, bright and bad for you

Refined white sugar, like white flour, has no nutritional value; all it does is to provide a quick-fix shot of energy in the form of simple carbohydrates. Most of the useful substances in sugar and flour have been extracted in the refining process. (Ironically, the nutritional part of the wheat is often repackaged as a 'health-giving' bran cereal.)

The problem with eating refined foods like this on a regular basis is not only that we fail to nourish our bodies properly, but we also run the risk of making ourselves ill. Many people today suffer from digestive disorders as a result of wheat or gluten intolerance, or from blood sugar problems (such as reactive hypoglycaemia), simply because our diets are based around too many refined carbohydrates – in particular, white sugar.

In the 21st century, we eat in two weeks the amount of sugar that our ancestors in the 18th century consumed in a year. This 2600 per cent increase has an enormous and far-reaching impact on our biochemistry. We were not designed for such a toxic load. Reduce it and health improves immediately.

This is scientifically documented. Researchers are clear about the fact that improving our diet, along the lines that we suggest in this book, can help to prevent long-term degenerative diseases, including cancer and heart disease.

**Genetically engineered (modified) foods**

For thousands of years, man has used the natural progression of change and development in agriculture. Sharp-eyed farmers and gardeners have always noticed which crops grew more robustly and produced a greater yield, choosing those strains for future production. The same principles have applied to farm animals, creating cows that are bigger, horses that are faster, and sheep that produce more wool. In comparison to the Middle Ages, for example, our agricultural output is increasingly plentiful. There is no harm in this type of agricultural science, largely because it involves natural selection and breeding to produce crops and animals that cater for changing needs and an ever-changing environment.

Genetically engineered (GE) foods, however, represent a radical departure from the natural process of change. Genetic engineering, also known as genetic modification (GM), involves the artificial insertion of a gene from one species into another. The technology has been in use for over 25 years, mainly in the pharmaceutical industry, but recently it has been applied to an increasing range of food crops and even animals. The purpose is to improve the recipient crop or animal in different ways, invariably for commercial reasons that are unrelated to nutrition and health. For example, genetic modification can make grain crops more resistant to pests, or give soft fruit a longer shelf life. To this end, human genes have been introduced into fish, for instance, and scorpion genes to tomatoes.

Although the supporters of GE technology (virtually all of whom have vested interests in it) vow that the procedure is safe and precise, many other independent experts say that this is simply untrue. There is no way of predicting exactly what the side-effects are, or what the long-term consequences of this vastly accelerated and unnatural process may be.

As animals, we are not adapted to deal with and dispose of engineered foods because we do not have a natural process of decoding these hybrid combinations and disposing of them from our systems. At present, we cannot recommend choosing any genetically engineered foods. For the record, no organic foods can be genetically engineered.

---

### Sweet treats

Puddings are definitely not off the menu, and you can choose from a variety of different options, according to the foods suggested on your Biotype diet. The following desserts are appropriate for all types.

- Fresh fruit
- Fruit Fool (see page 259)
- Fruit Dream (see page 260)
- Baked Apples with Fruit (see page 259)
- Red fruits (redcurrants, strawberries and raspberries – fresh or frozen), with 3 to 4 dessertspoons of sour cream, fromage frais, cottage cheese or yoghurt
- Cubed melon (any variety) in natural low-fat yoghurt with torn fresh mint and/or cinnamon
- Low-fat yoghurt with chopped fresh almonds and torn fresh mint
- Soaked stewed dried fruit, warm or cold, with sour cream, fromage frais, cottage cheese or yoghurt (substitute rhubarb in season, but not canned)
- Sliced water melon and kiwi (or other permitted fresh fruit), arrange overlapping slices on plate.

---

**Good-for-you grains**

Grains are the seeds and fruits of cereal grasses, filled with energy waiting to germinate into a plant. Whole-grains – made up of bran, germ, endo-and exosperms – are high in fibre, complex carbohydrates, vitamins and minerals. Refined grains, however, have been stripped of the bran and sometimes the germ. This process removes about 22 nutrients, some of which, perversely, must then be put back in a process misleadingly called 'enriching'. The bran is the outermost part of the grain; it contains B vitamins, proteins, fats and minerals and is a good source of fibre. The germ is rich in protein, polyunsaturated fatty acids, vitamins and minerals.

Spelt, faro and kamut are the ancient forms of wheat, grown in Egypt and Mediterranean countries. The Roman legions used these types of grain as a staple food for marching and fighting. These primitive grains have more protein and less gluten than their modern counterparts.

Quinoa, another ancient grain, was one of the most sacred foods of the Incas of South America, so nourishing, delicious and vital that they called it 'chesiya mama', or 'the Mother Grain'. The seeds are very nutritious, high in vitamin A, protein and fibre, and particularly rich in the amino acid lysine, as well as calcium, phosphorus and vitamins B and E.

With a basic understanding of healthy eating under your belt, it's now time to work out the diet that's right for your Biotype.

---

**Tip for all Types**

Put a glass of mineral water with a slice of lemon in it on your bedside table at night, so that you can have it as soon as you wake up in the morning. If you drink this in the night, make yourself another glass of hot water with a slice of lemon when you wake up. If you prefer cool water, squeeze the lemon so that you get some juice rather than just the flavour.

---

## Your Biotype diet

### Pathfinders

The basic philosophy of a Pathfinder diet is to stabilise the pituitary function and check the hormonal swings (caused by too much refined carbohydrate) of the adrenals and thyroid.

**Food to thrive on: a classic allergy diet**

Pathfinders function best on the classic 'low-allergen' diet: high in lean, low-fat protein (including poultry, fish and some red meat), salad and green vegetables, with some complex carbohydrates.

Pathfinders do not work well on foods that have been altered by man, such as refined carbohydrates (white sugar and white flour); you should also avoid gluten, milk and dairy products (except for butter and yoghurt).

## The Pathfinder way

Pathfinder Biotypes are dominated by the pituitary gland. You also invariably like dairy products such as ice-cream, milk and cheese. The problem is that this can set up a vicious cycle. The prolactin hormone in milk can over stimulate the pituitary, which can lead to more cravings for dairy foods. If you stick to a cycle of 'had some, want some more, had some, want some more', you are likely to suffer from arthritic conditions and overweight.

You also tend to go in cycles of ignoring food – you may easily go 24 hours without a bite, often on coffee and cigarettes – then overeat on high fat: 'Get me five chip butties with mayo, please.' What's more, those butties will go down without touching the sides: so Pathfinders can have a tendency to the digestive problems we discuss in Chapter 4.

As they age, Pathfinders tend to prefer bland food. The only illness to which this type often admits is a 'sensitive stomach'. Many bland foods are, of course, dairy based, which exacerbates any arthritic problems and tends to put on a soft podgy layer of watery fat.

Pathfinders have the highest metabolic rate and can both lose and gain weight incredibly quickly. In evolutionary terms, Pathfinders would have needed concentrated fuel to sustain that metabolic rate: rations like the Native American's favourite fast food, pemmican, which is a potent mix of ground up nuts, venison and fat. You need a constant supply of 'slow-burn' foods (see below), and should be certain to eat some protein (animal or vegetable) at every meal. Carbohydrates are allowed, but they should be complex, in the form of wholegrains, such as corn, wheat, barley, oats and so on, all with their outer shells. These casings contain vital nutrients, including vitamin E and essential fatty acids (EFAs).

Complex carbohydrates are more slowly absorbed, so they keep you going for longer. The difference between 'slow-burn' complex carbohydrates and 'fast-burn' junk food is exactly like the difference between setting light to a lump of coal or a sheet of paper.

Despite your indomitable will, you may find it hard to change your diet, by, for instance, raising your protein intake. A significant number of Pathfinders become vegetarians, and may go vegan, particularly when they're ill. If you are a vegetarian or vegan, you do need to be particularly careful to eat sufficient protein (see page 90). In fact, a high-carbohydrate diet will often weaken a Pathfinder because it puts the adrenals under constant assault and creates continual stress on the pituitary gland. It also has a knock-on effect, which suppresses the thyroid.

**Eat lots of**

Choose a variety of these foods on a rotating basis:
- Protein: chicken, guinea fowl, turkey and other poultry and game; oily fish, such as salmon, sea trout, tuna, mackerel, herring, sardines; veggie protein: tofu, tempeh and TVP (textured vegetable protein)
- Raw nuts and seeds: pine nuts, sunflower seeds, linseeds, pumpkin seeds, hazelnuts, almonds, walnuts
- Green vegetables that grow above the ground, 90 per cent cooked and 10 per cent raw

**Drink lots of**
- Mineral water
- Herbal teas

**Eat in moderation**

- Lean red meat (but not pork or pork products, except for the occasional organic ham or bacon treat)
- Whole-grains: brown rice, whole-wheat, whole-rye, oats, millet, barley, spelt, faro, kamut and quinoa
- Fresh fruits (avoid citrus fruits if you have an arthritic condition)
- Other vegetables, including carrots, garlic and onions, but excluding large tubers, such as potatoes, parsnips, swedes, turnips and celeriac
- Olive, corn and linseed oils
- Butter
- Live, natural yoghurt

**Drink in moderation**

- Organic decaffeinated coffee and tea (always water-washed, and organic; see page 47)
- Freshly made fruit juices, flavoured with herbs if you wish

**Try to avoid**

- Dairy products (except butter and natural yoghurt)
- Margarine
- Refined carbohydrates: all sugars (including galactose, glucose, maltose, sucrose, fructose and honey); white flour products such as cakes and biscuits, white bread, starches and starch thickeners
- Starch-heavy, large tubers, such as potatoes, parsnips, swedes, turnips and celeriac

**What to eat when**

Pathfinders do well on simple natural foods that have not been altered or processed by man. Typically, they are sensitive to diary products and refined products containing gluten (such as mass-produced bread, pasta, cakes, biscuits, pies, etc). Many supermarkets and healthfood stores now have a gluten-free section, which gives alternatives to most common gluten-containing products.

Pathfinders can eat protein at every meal. Remember this: breakfast like a king, lunch like a prince and dine like a pauper.

**Breakfast:**

Eat a substantial high protein meal with grains and/or nuts and seeds. For example, eggs, fish, poultry, whole-grain bread or crispbread, steak or organic meats.

**Menu ideas**

- Poached eggs with wholemeal toast
- Scrambled eggs and smoked salmon
- Kippers with bread and butter
- Poached undyed smoked haddock with bread and butter
- Cheese with rye bread
- Tofu fried in a little olive oil
- Classic Bircher Muesli (see page 261) with extra nuts and seeds soaked in apple or grape juice overnight; add sunflower, pumpkin and sesame seeds, almonds, hazelnuts, and walnuts
- Organic bacon and eggs with wholemeal toast

**Lunch:**

Eat a moderate meal with lean, low-fat protein, with green vegetables and salad. For example, poultry, oily fish, red meat or vegetable protein, with cooked green vegetables or a small salad, whole-grains such as brown rice, bread, or crisp bread, and a piece of fresh fruit.

**Menu ideas**

- Avocado with green salad
- Broccoli and mushroom salad with mixed nuts
- Smoked Tofu Salad (see page 251)
- Lamb steak with steamed vegetables
- Stir-fried fish with beansprouts and peppers
- Cold poached salmon with mushroom salad
- White fish (roasted or baked in parcel) with baked chicory or asparagus
- Beef steak with steamed vegetables
- Turkey steak/fillet with Mushroom and Fennel Salad (see page 245), or hot vegetables

**Supper:**

Eat the same type of meal as you did for lunch.

**Menu ideas**

- Soaked almonds (6 to 8) with cucumber and spring onion salad
- Grilled chicken with cauliflower and broccoli
- Roast venison with brown rice and green beans
- Pan-fried salmon with courgettes and herbs
- Chicken salad with pineapple and cucumber
- Baked tofu with Three Vegetable Mix (see page 258)
- Cold turkey slices with marinated carrot salad
- Roast vegetables with vegetarian parmesan shavings and olive oil
- Roast game: pheasant, partridge, grouse, etc., with wine gravy and vegetables
- Brown rice risotto
- Quinoa and cashew risotto
- Beetroots and quinoa with red cabbage

- Onions stuffed with quinoa, sundried tomatoes and anchovies
- Tahini, nut and vegetable rice salad
- Brown rice salad
- Mediterranean tofu casserole

## Hunter Gatherers

Of all the Biotypes, the Hunter Gatherers are the most sensitive to inappropriate eating. The aim of this diet, therefore, is to support the thyroid function and enhance its ability to perform its everyday tasks.

### Food to thrive on: a high-protein diet

Hunter Gatherers thrive on the food they would have had in the wild, gathered as they went on their nomadic way. Therefore, you will flourish on a diet that is high in lean, low-fat protein, with lots of vegetables and raw salads, fresh hard fruits and olive oil, and small amounts of whole-grain and wholemeal products. Crucial to Hunter Gatherer's health is a big breakfast to sustain you through the day.

You are more sensitive than the other Biotypes to the type of fats you eat, and should avoid dense saturated fats, such as animal fats (see page 127); you do well on foods containing a high level of unsaturated fats, such as olive oil and avocados.

Hunter Gatherers like to eat outside, so whenever possible have meals looking out on a view, on a balcony or in the garden; plan picnics and other open-air meals. At work, try to get out at lunchtime and go into a park or by a river.

## The Hunter Gatherer way

Imagine walking from your home to, say, the nearest town 50,000 years ago. Instead of roads and buildings, cars and lorries, you would pass over plains, alongside rivers and lakes, through woodland and dense forest, over hills and mountains. Every day, the Hunter Gatherers, both men and women, put on their buckskins, took up their spears and rucksack and went walkabout. Small wild animals were speared and stowed in the rucksack; greens, nuts, wild grains, fruits and seed heads would join them. In the evening, the Hunter Gatherers would gather round a fire and eat the raw foods and nuts. They would cook the hard-to-digest foods – meat, grains and seeds – in the embers overnight; by morning they would have a dense nutritious porridge and lean cooked meat. Once they had eaten, they would be off again. Lunch was left-over meat, supplemented with greens and fruit.

When the thyroid-dominant Hunter Gatherer is well and fit, your ample supply of thyroid hormones (which govern the metabolic rate) keep you naturally lithe and slim. You eat when you're hungry and never put on weight. But because of the delicate balance of this Biotype, Hunter Gatherers are particularly susceptible to gaining weight when stress throws that balance out of kilter and your metabolism becomes sluggish.

Hunter Gatherers tend to gain weight rapidly. It's often very obvious because this Biotype does not incorporate body fat neatly. Your slender wrists and ankles bear witness to the fact that however curvy your torso may become, you are designed by nature to be slim. Weight gain often occurs in women after childbirth; with men, work associated stress is the most common culprit. The weight gain won't always be due to thyroid dysfunction and its pear-shaped result. If the Hunter Gatherer has a strong metabolism, stress may thrust you into adrenal dys-function with its classic pattern of weight gain on your buttocks and belly.

Hunter Gatherers are particularly sensitive to any change of diet. Stress tends to make you look for quick-fix stimulants: sugar, chocolate, coffee, alcohol. You're the people who always fall for the 'naughty but nice' promise. In a rundown state, you find it hard to cope without stimulants and often get irritated at any suggestion of changing your diet.

In times of physical distress, going to the gym isn't the answer for this type; it will only stimulate the adrenal glands further. You need relaxation and rest coupled with gentle exercise in order to cope with reorganising your eating patterns.

**Eat lots of**

Choose a variety of these foods on a rotating basis:

- Proteins: eggs, poultry, fish particularly oily fish, such as herring, mackerel, sardines and salmon, or vegetable protein, such as tofu, tempeh or TVP
- Vegetables and fruit: choose mainly vegetables that grow above the ground and eat them in the form of salads. Choose hard fruits such as apples and pears. Eat 90 per cent cooked and 10 per cent raw

**Drink lots of**

- Mineral water
- Herbal teas

**Eat in moderation**

- Whole-grains: brown rice, wheat, rye, oats, spelt, faro, kamut and quinoa

- Corn, flaxseed and olive oils
- Butter
- Other fresh fruits
- Protein: organic meats and red meats (pork and bacon only if organic)

**Drink in moderation**
- Organic decaffeinated coffee and tea (always water-washed, and organic; see page 47)
- Freshly made fruit juices, flavoured with herbs if you wish

**Try to avoid**
- Refined carbohydrates: all sugars (including galactose, glucose, maltose, sucrose, fructose and honey); white flour products such as cakes and biscuits, white bread, starches and starch thickeners
- Deep- and shallow-fried foods (although food cooked in a wok is acceptable)
- Margarine
- Potatoes and other large starchy tubers, such as turnips, swedes, parsnips and celeriac
- Caffeinated coffee and tea, fizzy drinks, alcohol, fruit juices (except for freshly made juices; see above and page 187)

**What to eat when**
Hunter Gatherers are morning people; the worst thing you can do is skip a good breakfast (such as seed and nut muesli soaked overnight, eggs and organic bacon or kippers with organic whole-grain bread), which gives you stability. Snacks should be nuts and seeds, but if you eat well at each of your three main meals, you will be powered for a long day and need no extra.

**Breakfast:**

A substantial high-protein meal such as eggs, chicken, oily fish and/or whole-grain bread, crispbread, nut porridge or muesli.

**Menu ideas**

- Organic eggs and bacon, wholemeal or rye toast
- Organic bacon, with mushrooms and tomatoes, on toast
- Scrambled eggs and smoked salmon on rye or spelt toast
- Boiled egg/s with toast or bread and butter
- Classic Bircher Muesli (see page 261)
- Smoked haddock (undyed), poached in flavoured water, with soda bread
- Sardines on toast
- Kippers with bread and butter
- Soya yoghurt with mixed nuts and seeds
- Organic nut or peanut butter on wholemeal toast

**Lunch:**

Your midday meal should be light, with protein and vegetables or salad. For example, cheese, red meat, poultry, oily fish, and vegetable protein, with as many vegetables as you like, or salad.

**Menu ideas**

- Grilled chicken with green vegetables
- Chicken roasted with olive oil and wine and herbs, with sliced deseeded red and yellow peppers and courgette chunks roasted with the bird
- Grilled lemon sole or any other fish, with spinach and toasted pine nuts
- Fish portions baked in a parcel with seasonal vegetables
- Roasted salmon or cod portions with lemon olive oil and courgettes

- Californian style brochettes (see page 231)
- Pan-fried turkey fillets with broccoli
- Stir-fried vegetables
- Roasted vegetables topped with goat's cheese or parmesan shavings
- Vegetarian sausages and green beans topped with toasted flaked almonds

**Supper:**
Eat much the same type of meal as you did at lunch, adding hard fruits.

**Menu ideas**
- Avocado with green salad and sprouted grains
- Big bowl of fruit salad with nuts and natural yoghurt, if wished
- Smoked tofu in broth with seasonal greens
- Cauliflower salad
- Smoked Tofu Salad (see page 251)
- Crudités with hummus, guacamole, tzatziki (don't hesitate to buy the dips)

---

**Bread**

Many people believe that bread is made of wheat flour. Well, that's certainly true, but it's not the whole truth. Modern wheat seems to disagree with lots of people's stomachs and there are lots of alternatives available in your supermarket and healthfood store, starting with rye bread and pumpernickel, which suit most people. So look around for non-wheat, or part-wheat loaves.

Also look for loaves made with the ancient forms of wheat, such as kamut and spelt, which are much less likely to cause

---

---

sensitivity. Kamut and spelt are also used for pasta and other products traditionally made of wheat flour. Also try oat cakes and rice cakes, which are delicious alternatives to bread.

---

## Pioneers

The aim of the Pioneer diet is to deliver a stable food pattern that supports rather than taxes the adrenal gland. Reducing physical stress in this way enables the Pioneer to keep going, and going, and going . . .

### Food to thrive on: food-combining

Pioneers do well on simple meals that follow the principles of food-combining. As well as being more suitable for your metabolism, food-combining often proves the simplest way for Pioneers to lose weight. The system is based on separating proteins and carbohydrates at main meals, and eating fruit on its own (see panel, page 70).

Pioneers often ignore where they eat, so a sandwich at a desk, while talking on the phone, is the norm. In fact, because you do well in situations where structure is imposed on you, and usually enjoy eating as a form of relaxation, you tend to like the ritual of eating out in a favourite restaurant or café. You have to sit down peacefully for a given period of time, choose from a list of possible dishes, and wait until they appear – all of which is soothing for the Pioneer temperament.

## The Pioneer way

This way of eating developed as a survival technique. Imagine the Pioneers in their covered wagons, rolling across the prairies or veldt for months at a time. With no time to grow food crops, they were reliant on food that was highly nutritious, compact, easily transportable and non-perishable, supplemented by what could be gleaned from the land when the wagons rolled to a full stop for the evening. If the men shot game, the wagon train would eat it in a variety of different ways, with greens found along the journey. In other words, their diet consisted of protein and vegetables. When neither was available, they would rely on pulses – like baked beans – and bread. That's why food-combining – where protein and starch meals are separated – suits Pioneer types.

Eating in this manner is admirably adapted to survival (brilliant for the castaways who seem to people our TV screens nowadays). There's not a lot of variety, but that doesn't usually bother Pioneer types. They eat the same meals contentedly day after day. 'What's for lunch? Oh, coconuts again? Grated or cubed? Well, that's nice.'

Nowadays, of course, Pioneers can consume in one day a variety of foods that they would never have had the chance of eating in weeks and months. So it need not be boring – unless, of course, the Pioneer is a man cooking for himself, when it might well be.

Pioneers are slow metabolisers. Along with the Farmer Gardeners, you are the slowest to burn body fat which gives you balance and stability. Pioneers often develop body fat as a response to stress but, conversely, you can lose weight on holiday (that means resting and relaxing – not vegging out on the sofa with a curry and a lager).

## The basic principles of food-combining

- Don't mix foods and food products in the left-hand column below with foods in the right-hand column.
- Always eat fruit at least 30 minutes on either side of meals.

| Proteins | Starches |
|---|---|
| Beef | Barley, bulgar, corn, millet, oats, rye, wheat, quinoa |
| Canned fish | Biscuits, bread, buns, cakes |
| Cheese | Flour, all kinds |
| Chicken | Muesli |
| Eggs | Pasta |
| Fish | Pastry |
| Game | Potatoes, sweet potatoes, yams |
| Lamb | Pulses (except soya) |
| Pork | Rice |
| Shellfish | Soya beans and soya milk |
| TVP (textured vegetable protein) | Tofu, beancurd |
| Turkey | |

### Eat lots of

Choose a variety of these foods on a rotating basis:

- Whole-grains and grain products: brown rice, rye, barley, oats, buckwheat, millet, whole-wheat, spelt, faro, kamut (as they are, or made into bread, pasta or pancakes), quinoa
- Pulses: beans, lentils, peas, chick peas, tofu, tempeh, TVP

- Vegetables and salads in season: particularly green vegetables, raw salads, root vegetables, chicory and all bitter leaves, and tomatoes
- Fruits in season, but avoid bananas and grapes totally

**Drink lots of**
- Still mineral water
- Herbal teas

**Eat in moderation**
- Fish: particularly oily fish, such as salmon, mackerel, herrings, sardines, tuna, and white fish
- Poultry: without skin
- Eggs: no more than three a week
- Olive, corn and flaxseed oils
- Raw nuts and seeds: buy unshelled and unroasted
- Potatoes
- Organic cow's or goat's milk butter
- Organic full-fat cow's, goat's or sheep's milk
- Organic cow's, goat's or sheep's milk plain yoghurt

**Drink in moderation**
- Organic decaffeinated coffee and tea (always water-washed, and organic; see page 47)
- Freshly made fruit juices, flavoured with herbs if you wish

**Try to avoid**
- Salt and salty foods
- Red meat
- Pork and pork products (an occasional organic bacon or ham treat is acceptable)
- Shellfish

- Deep-fried foods (fry lightly in a spoonful of olive oil, if necessary)
- Cheese
- Margarine
- Refined carbohydrates: all sugars (including galactose, glucose, maltose, sucrose, fructose and honey); white flour products such as cakes and biscuits, white bread, starches and starch thickeners
- Caffeinated drinks, including coffee, tea and cola
- Fizzy carbonated drinks
- Alcohol (see Treats)

### What to eat when

Aim to build up your meals during the day so that breakfast is lighter than lunch, and lunch lighter than your substantial dinner.

The Pioneer Biotype diet is based on food-combining. That's a slightly confusing term because it means separating protein meals from starch meals. So, for instance, you might fancy a boiled egg for breakfast but you shouldn't have it with bread and butter. Equally you could have toast, but not with bacon.

As a rule of thumb, fruit is generally better separated from protein and starch meals and eaten as a snack, but you can have a fruit-based meal, where you combine any fruit with salad or raw vegetables, natural yoghurt, nuts (almonds, hazelnuts, brazil nuts and pine nuts), sunflower and pumpkin seeds. Melon is best eaten separately from other foods, except natural yoghurt.

Food-combining may sound confusing but you very quickly get used to it. Here is an easy to follow chart.

## Which foods to combine

| Protein foods | Neutral foods | Starch foods |
|---|---|---|
| Meat | Vegetables (not potatoes) | Bread |
| Fish | Salads | Pasta |
| Cheese | Fats and oils (including butter and cream) | Potatoes |
| Eggs | Cream cheese | Rice |
| Dairy products | Herbs and spices *Also*, but eat in small quantities: raisin, nuts and seeds | Grains |
| *Combine with:* any vegetables except potatoes Salad | *Combine with:* either protein *or* starch | *Combine with:* any vegetables salad any nuts and seeds pulses butter, cream and natural cream cheese |

See also Vegetarian section (page 90).

**Breakfast:**

Breakfast should be a light meal, with fruit and grain products. For example, whole-grain or whole-wheat bread or crisp-bread, sugar-free muesli, dried fruit, porridge, fresh fruit or yoghurt.

On the whole, Pioneers do better with a light breakfast, a more substantial lunch and dinner that is larger than lunch. However, this is flexible so choose your breakfast according to your individual need and inclination.

**Menu ideas**

Starch (carbohydrate):
- 3 pieces of fresh fruit, any kind
- Dried fruit soaked overnight in fruit juice (apple, pear, grape), topped with Greek yoghurt
- Puffed grain cereal with soya milk
- Porridge made with coconut milk
- Breakfast Summer Pudding (see page 262)
- Mushrooms and tomatoes on toast
- Muesli (see recipes) with unsweetened soya milk and/or a blob of organic cow's cream, if you like
- Porridge with raisins and organic honey, plus full-fat cream, if wished
- Sugar-free breakfast cereals with soya milk, plus organic dairy cream, if wished
- Fruit salad (no melon) with chopped mixed nuts, honey and natural live yoghurt, plus whole-grain toast and fruit spread

Protein (these are heavier options, so don't have too much):
- Eggs and bacon (must be organic)
- Scrambled eggs with smoked salmon or tomato
- Poached eggs and spinach

- Smoked haddock, poached in milk
- Kippers

**Lunch:**
Eat a more substantial lunch, with vegetables, salad and grain products. For example, steamed vegetables, anything whole-grain (see page 55), and fresh fruit.

**Menu ideas**
Starch (carbohydrate) – light lunches or starters:
- Asparagus or artichokes hot with lemon butter or mayo
- Avocado, leeks, tomato and basil vinaigrette
- Peppers roast and peeled, with olive oil and shaved parmesan
- Vegetable soup (try roast tomatoes and roasted. skinned red peppers liquidised with stock and herbs, hot or cold, and topped with fromage frais and pesto or tapenade)

Protein – light lunches or starters:
- Fresh shell-on prawns with homemade mayo
- Parma ham with ripe pears and/or mango and/or figs
- Cauliflower salad with Vogel bread
- Cucumber and spring onion salad with chickpeas or hummus
- Marinated carrot salad or pineapple and cucumber salad with brown rice (hot or cold)
- Spinach salad with pumpernickel
- Avocado and green salad
- Corn on the cob with bean sprout salad

Starch (carbohydrates) – larger lunches:
- Risotto or pasta with herbs, fungi, tomatoes, etc., with olive oil and butter (see Quinoa Risotto, page 232) but no parmesan (try vegetarian if you want, or cream cheese)

- Jacket potato, with baked beans (sugar-free) and salad
- Sandwich made with whole-grain bread and organic butter or olive oil, with avocado and salad

Protein – larger lunches:
- Serve with vegetable crisps if wished (not potato crisps; and no potatoes in these protein menus)
- Plain grilled fish, chicken, lamb or beef (organic) with vegetables and salad
- Caesar salad (no bread croutons) with chopped fried bacon, chicken or tuna
- Smoked trout fillets with mango slices and watercress salad with vinaigrette
- Omelette 'fines herbes', with cheese, tomato or mushroom
- Grilled king prawns with salad or vegetable stir fry
- Crab salad with avocado and artichoke hearts
- Tricolore salad: tomato, mozzarella and avocado with basil, olive oil and balsamic vinegar or lemon

**Supper:**

Go for a bigger supper, with protein or grains, vegetables, salad and fruit. For example, poultry or fish, beans such as haricots, butter beans or lentils, vegetables and fruit. Choose one of the lunch options as starters or for a lighter dinner.

**Menu ideas**

Starch (carbohydrate):
- Choose any of the lunch options, and follow with fruit.
- Pasta with pesto, roasted peppers and pine nuts, with salad
- Mushroom risotto with cucumber and tomato salad
- Ciabatta topped with tomatoes, basil, pine nuts, sundried

tomatoes and red onions, grilled (bruschetta)
- Baked potato with ratatouille, with a salad
- Garlic and rosemary mashed potatoes, topped with stir-fried tomatoes, courgettes, onions, garlic, peppers and aubergine, topped with torn basil and lots of black pepper
- Paul's Root Vegetable Stew (see page 257), served with warm herb foccacia

Protein:
Serve with fresh vegetables or salad; follow with cheese. Alternatively, choose any of the lunch options.
- Oysters, smoked salmon, trout, eel or dressed crab
- Scallops with asparagus, or Thai-style with soy and ginger and stir-fried leaves
- Fish soup with rouille
- Grilled game hen or quail with courgette chunks, asparagus, artichoke hearts and fresh peas, cooked in olive oil and white wine and finished with lots of chopped fresh mint
- Tarragon chicken, make sauce with juices and cream, if wished
- Roast duck, or duck breasts, served pink with green pepper sauce
- Rack of lamb with garlic and rosemary
- Seared tuna with tapenade blended briefly with coriander leaves and roasted garlic (popped out of skins)
- Whole small sea bass stuffed with herbs (or trout)
- Roast cod with mustard topping and meat jus
- Salmon, hot or cold, with green mayonnaise
- Fillet of beef, plain or stuffed with pate and olives

> **Note**
>
> Some Pioneers do better with more protein, vegetable and salad meals, rather than alternating them with starches.

### Farmer Gardeners

Farmer Gardeners tend to have high levels of the reproductive hormones oestrogen and testosterone, and are prone to swings in these. A lacto-vegetarian diet creates a state of hormonal balance at the same time as increasing the rate at which food is metabolised (turned into energy) in the body.

#### Food to thrive on: a lacto-vegetarian diet

Like the Pioneers, Farmer Gardeners tend to be slow metabolisers, so you need light foods that will provide instant energy and take little time to digest. You should avoid spicy food such as curries.

Translate that into a diet and it means that Farmer Gardeners do well on a lacto-vegetarian diet. As well as dairy products, you should eat lots of vegetables, salads and fruits daily, with smaller amounts of whole-grain products. It's essential that this Biotype eats small amounts of protein (animal, fish or vegetarian) at lunch time, but you are the only Biotype that can thrive on a vegan diet.

Farmer Gardeners are convivial folk who enjoy company while they're preparing and eating food. They also tend to like familiar surroundings, so the kitchen table is a perfect place to eat — whether it's their own or someone else's.

## The Farmer Gardener way

Farmer Gardeners are the original settlers who chose not to move on with the Pioneers (often the type of person you are found with today), or to look over the horizon. Most Farmer Gardeners have an amazing ability to be content and happy where they are.

You are curious, but it's not about knowing what's on the other side of the mountain; rather, you are interested in knowing about what's in front of you. Once it would mostly have been plants and soil parasites. Now it includes anything that's in your immediate environment – house, community or office.

Farmers are suited to live off what they could have grown on smallholdings – mostly simple, seasonal foodstuffs such as beans, grains and seasonal vegetables and fruit. They also dined on what they could make from small farm animals, such as goats or sheep. Some items were fresh, others were dried or preserved. Some locally-caught fish, poultry and game would supplement their diet but, unlike the Hunter Gatherers, Farmer Gardeners wouldn't go on hunting expeditions, which might involve a trip to the other side of the mountain.

**Eat lots of**
- Dairy products: cheeses, hard and soft (goat's or sheep's, preferably)
- Goat's and sheep's yoghurt
- Full-fat organic milk
- Other dairy products, such as quark and creme frâiche (but not butter or cream)
- Green and root vegetables, salads, endive and Chinese leaves

- Fruit: apples, pears, soft fruits, dates, figs, exotic fruits
- Whole-grains and grain products: brown rice, rye, barley, oats, buckwheat, millet, wheat, spelt, farro, quinoa, and kamut (as they are, or made into bread, pasta or pancakes)

**Drink lots of**
- Mineral water
- Herbal teas

**Eat in moderation**
- Oily fish: mackerel, herrings, kippers, pilchards, trout, salmon, sardines, fresh tuna, anchovies
- Poultry: chicken, turkey, guinea fowl
- Corn, linseed and olive oils
- Eggs: no more than three a week
- Nuts and seeds: hazel nuts, almonds, walnuts, pine nuts, sunflower seeds, linseeds, pumpkin seeds

**Drink in moderation**
- Organic decaffeinated coffee and tea (always water-washed, and organic; see page 47)
- Freshly made fruit juices, flavoured with herbs if you wish

**Try to avoid**
- Red meat
- Pork and pork products (except for the occasional organic ham or bacon treat)
- Spices
- Cream and ice-cream
- Fried and/or oily foods
- Butter and margarine

- Refined carbohydrates: all sugars (including galactose, glucose, maltose, sucrose, fructose and honey); white flour products such as cakes and biscuits, white bread, starches and starch thickeners
- Non-organic, caffeinated coffee and tea (see above)
- Alcohol (see page 46)
- Fizzy drinks

**What to eat when**
The Farmer Gardener is ideally suited to produce that's grown or raised locally. Living off the farm or kitchen garden is the ideal. In default of this, try and shop for locally grown food and eat seasonally, where possible. The lacto (dairy) component is a prime source of protein for the Farmer Gardener, so you should try to include a dairy-based component to one of your meals every day.

Breakfast and lunch are light; the evening meal is more substantial.

**Breakfast:**
A meal based around fruit and grains; for example, fresh or soaked, dried and unsulphured fruits, yoghurt, whole-grain breads and cereals, or crispbread.

**Menu ideas**
- Soaked dried fruit with yoghurt
- Classic Bircher Muesli (see page 261) with fresh fruit (such as peaches, pears, plums, kiwi, etc)
- Breakfast Summer Pudding (see page 262)
- Breakfast Muffins (see page 263)
- Natural yoghurt with flaked soaked almonds
- Soya yoghurt with seasonal fruits

- Rye bread/pumpernickel and cream cheese/cottage cheese
- Wholemeal nut loaf with Marmite

**Lunch:**

Include a small amount of light protein (such as fish, poultry or a vegetable protein), and grains, along with plenty of vegetables and/or salad.

**Menu ideas**

- Tricolore salad: avocado, mozzarella, tomatoes
- Fennel and mushroom salad with 2oz (50g) walnuts or almonds
- Sprouted bean salad with rye bread/pumpernickel and cream cheese/cottage cheese
- Tofu in broth, with hot greens
- Three-bean salad with wholemeal bread
- Roasted root vegetables with parmesan shavings
- Grilled goat's cheese with green salad dressed with walnut oil and crumbled walnuts
- Trout, baked in a parcel, with seasonal vegetables or a salad
- Grilled or tinned sardines
- Classic Caesar salad with anchovies
- Salmon brochettes with peppers and mushrooms
- Turkey steak with seasonal vegetables or a salad
- Grilled chicken breast/drumsticks (hot or cold) with salad
- Cheese and asparagus pancakes with mozzarella/goat's cheese (make buckwheat pancakes, fold round cooked asparagus, lay overlapping slices of mozzarella or goat's cheese on top and slip under the grill until bubbling)
- Greek salad (tomatoes, feta, black olives, cucumber)
- Nicoise salad

**Dinner:**

Dinner should be a more substantial meal, including salad, vegetables and either a whole-grain product or a small amount of light protein.

**Menu ideas**

- Brown rice risotto or salad with herbs and soaked nuts, and a green salad
- Whole-grain penne (spelt or kamut) with tomato and basil sauce and parmesan, if wished
- Whole-grain spaghetti with roast tomato and roast red pepper sauce and parmesan, if wished
- Whole-grain taglierini with peas, asparagus and crème fraîche or Greek yoghurt
- Peppers stuffed with savoury rice, and a salad
- Quinoa risotto, with herbs, fresh vegetables in season
- Brown rice risotto with seasonal vegetables
- Beetroot and quinoa with red cabbage; stewed dried fruit with fromage frais
- Omelette with herbs and sorrel, tomato salad
- Marrow stuffed with rice, served with tomato sauce

---

**Top tip**

You can heat Greek style yoghurt as long as you heat it gently in a heatproof bowl over a pan of simmering water. Don't boil it!

---

### Dancers

Dancers, with their combination of glandular influences (the pituitary and the gonads), have the strengths of both the Pathfinder and the Farmer Gardener. This diet is designed to maintain an even balance between the two interdependent glands, which allows both to function at optimum level.

#### Food to thrive on: a demi-vegetarian diet

Dancers flourish on a demi-vegetarian diet – in keeping with your adaptable nature. This diet is truly eclectic, containing elements of all the food groups. The Dancer can break many of the 'rules', such as not eating fruit at the end of a meal and avoiding gluten and dairy produce.

Although the basis of this eating plan is very similar to the diet for Farmer Gardeners, Dancers have a slightly faster metabolism than Farmer Gardeners and need more 'slow-burn' food (such as seeds and nuts). For lunch every day, you must have lean protein, such as chicken, turkey, guinea fowl and fish, or veggie protein, such as tofu, to avoid suffering a mid-afternoon dip.

You will not do well on the Farmer Gardeners' lacto-vegetarian (or vegan) diet, although you can, of course, substitute vegetarian protein for animal on any occasion. Dancers should be careful to restrict cow's milk products, such as ice-cream and cheese, because they have the Path-finders' problems with pituitary function and dairy foods, which can lead eventually to arthritic conditions and over-weight. Usually, however, they can eat sheep's and goat's milk products without problems.

## The Dancer way

The Dancer Biotype may be urban, but all things are relative. Remember that you emerged from herding people, not from a burger and shake bar. Dancers came from an agrarian society where grains, crops and farmed animal protein – cows, goats, sheep – were all established and available.

Dancers tend to choose meals on the indulgence principle: lunch at your desk might be a box of handmade truffles and an apple (which makes it healthy). At a restaurant you might well have three starters and a good proportion of the dessert trolley.

Dancers tend to have a compulsive streak, like the Pathfinders, so inherit that type's craving for dairy products; ice-cream seems to be a frequent food dream. You also tend to think – mistakenly – that you have the Pathfinders' strength and endurance. So you're inclined, for instance, to skip meals – a big mistake for any type – or resort to quick fixes, such as vitamin B12 injections (we know Geri Halliwell does it but we don't support those, either). You are, however, the only type that can get by with a meal at the desk – as long as you do eat it and it's sensible.

Dancers don't do long-term planning. You are delightful hosts and the meal will be beautifully presented, but casseroles won't be on the menu unless you've bought them in. There's absolutely nothing wrong with this, so pander to your nature and opt for quick-fix food.

**Eat lots of**

Choose a variety of these foods on a rotating basis:
- Dairy products: cheeses, hard and soft (preferably goat's or

sheep's); yoghurt (goat's and sheep's); full fat organic milk; other dairy products, such as quark and crème fraîche (but not butter or cream)

- Whole-grains and grain products: brown rice, rye, barley, oats, buckwheat, millet, wheat, spelt, farro, quinoa and kamut (as they are, or made into bread, pasta or pancakes)
- Green and root vegetables, salads, endive, Chinese leaves
- Fruit: apples, pears, soft fruits, dates, figs, exotic fruits

**Drink lots of**
- Mineral water
- Herbal teas

**Eat in moderation**
- Fish of all kinds, particularly oily fish such as mackerel, herrings, kippers, pilchards, trout, salmon, sardines, fresh tuna, anchovies
- Poultry: chicken, turkey, guinea fowl
- Eggs: no more than three a week
- Olive, corn and linseed oils
- Nuts and seeds: pine nuts, sunflower seeds, linseeds, pumpkin seeds, hazel nuts, almonds, walnuts

**Drink in moderation**
- Fruit juices, especially apple, pear, peach, berries and soft fruits
- Organic decaffeinated coffee and tea (always water-washed, and organic; see page 47)

**Try to avoid**
- Red meat
- Pork and pork products (the occasional organic treat is OK)

- Spices and spicy foods
- Cream, especially ice-cream
- Fried and/or oily foods
- Butter and margarine
- Refined carbohydrates: all sugars (including galactose, glucose, maltose, sucrose, fructose and honey); white flour products, such as cakes and biscuits, white bread, starches and starch thickeners
- Non-organic, caffeinated coffee and tea (see above)
- Alcohol (see page 46)
- Colas and other fizzy drinks

**What to eat when**

The Dancer is the truly adapted specimen of modern mankind. Their small stature and relatively fast metabolic rate means that they can tolerate just about every kind of food as long as it is in moderation: they have virtually no tendencies toward food sensitivities. The Dancer can be vegetarian or eat meat, food-combine or the opposite, with little or no impact on their health. They do, however, need to be careful of cow's milk products, as we mentioned earlier, because of their inherited susceptibility to dairy craving and arthritis.

The secret to a healthy Dancer diet is rotating the different food types from day to day: vegetarian, high-protein, food-combining. Always remember to have some form of protein (animal or vegetarian) at lunch.

As with every person, regardless of type, Dancers need to learn to listen to their bodies and respond with the food that suits them best at any particular time.

Aim to make breakfast and lunch light, and dinner more substantial

**Breakfast:**

Breakfast should be a light meal, with fruit and grain. Choose from fresh or soaked, dried, unsulphured fruit, yoghurt, wholegrain breads or cereals and crispbread.

**Menu ideas**

- Yoghurt and fresh fruit, mixed with 2 tbsp (30ml) of muesli base
- Soya yoghurt with soaked seeds: soak sunflower, pumpkin and sesame seeds overnight in apple or orange juice
- Puffed grain cereal with milk, topped with grated apple tossed in lemon juice
- Stewed mixed fruit mixed into muesli, made with fruit juice
- Classic Bircher Muesli (see page 261)
- Porridge made from oat groats, topped with stewed fruit
- 3 pieces of fresh fruit, and toast with cream cheese
- Fresh fruit salad with yoghurt
- Fruit smoothie (liquidise fruit with thin natural yoghurt, such as live goat's yoghurt)
- Breakfast Muffins (see page 263)
- Breakfast Summer Pudding (see page 262)

**Lunch:**

Another light meal, with a small amount of protein, plus salad and/or vegetables, and grains. Choose from fish, poultry, eggs or vegetable proteins, and add plenty of vegetables and/or salad.

**Menu ideas**

- Tofu with rice, green salad or vegetables
- Onions stuffed with sundried tomatoes, quinoa and anchovies

- Steamed or grilled white fish with spinach (hot or as salad) or other green vegetable; wholemeal bread
- Roast cod with green vegetables and puy lentils
- Salad Nicoise
- Cold salmon with Mushroom and Fennel Salad (see page 245)
- Smoked mackerel fillet (fresh mackerel, if available) with gooseberry sauce (use frozen if not in season), watercress salad and oatcakes
- Salmon mayonnaise with wholemeal bread and salad (easy sandwich)
- Organic bacon, mushroom and tomatoes with whole-grain toast
- Fishcakes with spinach, or other green vegetables
- Sardines on rye toast with tomatoes and watercress
- Grilled Dover or lemon sole with pilau rice and fennel salad
- Poached undyed smoked haddock, with puréed root vegetables (such as carrot and celeriac)
- Organic proscuitto with pears, mango and/or figs, plus watercress with olive oil and bread
- Grilled chicken with butter/olive oil and balsamic vinegar, green vegetables and/or salad, wholemeal bread
- Chicken broth with vegetables and rice pasta (or spelt or kamut pasta), all mixed in
- Fish broth
- Mussels with fromage frais and tarragon
- Tomato, bean and bacon stew

**Dinner:**

Dinner should be a more substantial meal, with vegetables and some form of protein, as well as some fruit. For example, eggs, poultry, fish, or vegetable proteins, with vegetables, salad and fruit to finish.

**Menu ideas**

- Mange Tout and Avocado Salad (see page 242)
- Caribbean Salad (see page 247), goat's milk cheese and celery with oatcakes
- Cauliflower salad with 2oz (50g) walnuts
- Roast vegetables with shaved parmesan, wholemeal bread, goat's cheese and fruit
- Vegetable stew with brown rice, Fruit Dream (see page 260)
- Gado-gado (see page 248), fruit salad
- Quinoa risotto, with mushrooms and herbs, or peas and courgettes, and fruit
- Brown rice risotto with seasonal vegetables
- Beetroot and quinoa with red cabbage
- Spicy lentil bake with green leaf salad
- Split pea or lentil soup (cooked with a ham bone if you're not vegetarian)
- Pasta (whole-grain, rice, spelt or kamut, preferably) with roast tomato and basil sauce, cheese and fruit

---

## Guidelines for vegetarians

Eating lots of fruit and vegetables is a wonderful way to kick-start your wellbeing programme, and they are proven both to help keep you healthy and to prevent disease. However, the decision to adopt a vegetarian diet (which involves cutting out meat, poultry and fish) or a vegan regime (eating only plant-based products) should be considered carefully. You may be at risk of missing some of the essential nutrients (in particular, protein, iron and vitamin B12), and these are crucial to health and wellbeing on all levels. For this reason, we strongly suggest that anyone under the age of 18 does not adopt a vegan diet.

In order to make up for these deficiencies, some vegetarian diets recommend eating lots of carbohydrates. This does make up the shortfall, but also tends to pile on the pounds. So, for vegetarians and most particularly vegans, it's important to spend a little while understanding the situation and planning your meals. In some cases, it's also wise to take a supplement, in the form of a proprietary product or as an extra helping of a particular food every day.

It's also vital to choose fresh, organically produced foods. Because modern industrial farming techniques rely heavily on the use of synthetic nitrogen-based fertilisers instead of the more traditional farming techniques (such as crop rotation, animal fertiliser, fallow fields and straight forward mulch and manure), the soil itself has been depleted of essential nutrients. It follows that the food produced from this soil is also depleted. Food crops are only as good as the soil in which they are grown, and this is something that many consumers are not told. The more organic food you incorporate in your diet, the better. A vegetarian eating only conventionally produced foods will need to eat more to get enough basic nutrients.

## Potential problems and solutions

### Problem 1: Protein and amino acids

Proteins are made of amino acids. There are 20 in all, of which eight – the so-called essential amino acids – cannot be made by our bodies and must come from our diet. 'Complete protein', which has all eight amino acids, is found in meat and fish. No single plant food is complete, however, so the amino acids must come from combinations of a grain and one or more plants.

Vegetarians who eat eggs and cheese will invariably get the eight amino acids. Eggs, for example, are regarded as a 'perfect food' in terms of complete protein. But vegans, especially those trying to lose weight, need to take special care to get all eight. Pregnant and breastfeeding mothers should also be certain they are getting all the necessary nutrients.

The following symptoms are associated with too little protein:

- loss of energy
- lack of stamina
- depression
- poor resistance to infection
- physical weakness in the shape of weak arms and legs, associated with a reduced ability to walk and run, plus general tiredness
- loss of hair and/or hair colour
- swelling of joints
- increased sensitivity to the cold

**Solution:**
It was once believed that you needed to have complete protein – the eight essential amino acids – at every meal. However, recent research from the Vegetarian Society has shown that these amino acids can exist in your body a little bit longer than was thought. So you need to plan your meals so that you get plenty of the essential amino acids on a *daily* basis.

Anyone who is leading a very active life – working out or training, for instance – should consider taking an amino acid supplement, such as Broad Spectrum Amino Acids by Biocare.

Good sources of 'complete' vegetarian proteins include:
- free-range organically produced eggs
- dairy products, including cheese, whole milk and yoghurt (butter and cream are poor sources of protein)
- soya products, including tofu, tempeh, textured vegetable protein, veggie burgers, soya milk
- quorn

*Making a complete vegetarian protein*
Using the list below, combine one of the basic foods on the left, with one or more of the other foods in the right-hand column.

| Basic food | Serve with |
| --- | --- |
| Rice | Beans, peas, lentils, nuts, salad, raw vegetables |
| Wholemeal bread | Nut butter and tahini, beans, tofu, lentil soup, pea soup |
| Raw vegetables and salad | Rice, millet, mushrooms, brazil nuts, sesame seeds, tahini |
| Peanuts | Nuts, sunflower seeds, pumpkin seeds |
| Oats | Soya milk, nuts, seeds |
| Wholewheat cereals | Soya milk, nuts, seeds |
| Millet | Beans, peas, lentils, nuts, seeds, raw vegetables, salad, soya milk, tofu |
| Potato | Soya milk |
| Sweetcorn | Beans |

*Top tips for a vegetarian diet:*

- Chick peas and baked beans are great sources of veggie protein
- Eat five almonds for breakfast. Soak almonds for 24 hours at room temperature, not in the fridge. According to the Ayurvedic medical tradition from India, leaving the almonds for that time allows them to germinate so that the oil in the endosperm of the nut is converted into easily digested vegetable protein.
- If you prefer not to use cow's milk, try soya, oat, rice or almond milk (available in healthfood stores and good supermarkets)

### Problem 2: Vitamin B12 and iron

B12 is a helper vitamin, involved in the utilisation of amino acids, vitamins B5 and C, folic acid and also iron. If people lack the ability to absorb vitamin B12, or do not consume enough, they run the risk of pernicious anaemia (the type of anaemia associated with lack of B12, as opposed to lack of iron; although the cause is different, the effect is the same, see below).

There are two problems for vegetarians: B12 is not present in plant foods and iron is not as easily absorbed from vegetable sources as it is from animal.

The following symptoms are associated with vitamin B12 deficiency:

- nervousness
- neuritis (nerve pain – often in the form of tiny 'electric shocks')
- numbness of fingers and toes
- poor muscular coordination
- unpleasant body odour
- PMS (pre-menstrual syndrome)

The following symptoms are associated with iron deficiency:
- because iron is associated with the transport of oxygen in the blood, people suffering from anaemia often suffer dizziness on physical exertion
- palpitations
- fatigue
- headache
- insomnia
- pale to very pale skin, lips and inner eyelids

**Solution:**

To reduce the risk of vitamin B12 deficiency, vegetarians who eat dairy products and eggs should ensure they have a daily intake of one or other of these so that they get the small amount of B12 they need.

Vegans and vegetarians eating few animal foods should take a B12 supplement or include B12-fortified foods into their diet; for example, yeast extracts (Marmite is vegan and contains B12), soya milk, veggie burgers, some breakfast cereals.

To prevent iron deficiency, take a dessertspoonful of black-strap molasses daily and ensure that you eat plenty of fruit and vegetables for their vitamin C content. Vitamin C is required for iron to be properly absorbed by the body. As well as fresh fruit and vegetables (particularly leafy green vegetables), eat dried apricots and figs, plus lentils and other pulses, and wholemeal bread.

Floradix liquid iron and vitamin formula (yeast- and gluten-free), by Floravital is a useful supplement.

# The Effects of Stress: Detecting and Correcting Stress Weaknesses

As we explained earlier, the stresses and strains of modern life affect many of us, particularly in the West. Even if the problems are not serious, they can significantly impair your quality of life. The checklists below are designed to help you detect any weak points, and correct them with the help of nutrition and other natural supports, so that you feel your best at all times.

This advice does not, of course, replace a consultation with an expert. If you have any doubts about your health, or specific questions that you need answered, please consult a doctor or other qualified health professional. Equally, if simple shifts don't improve your daily life, we suggest you talk to a life coach or counsellor (see page 277).

When you go through the Stress Weakness checklists you will see that the format for scoring is the same for each one. If you score zero, you obviously don't need to do anything. But if, like most of us, you identify some weaknesses, you will find that there are three problem zones: scores of 1 to 8, 9 to 20, and 20 upwards.

For scores of 1 to 8, there is a Basic Stress Weakness Programme (see page 98) to strengthen and correct all the stress points; this begins with your individual Biotype diet. There is also a specific Supplement Programme for each problem, which is recommended for anyone scoring between 9 and 20. If you score more than 20, we advise you to consult your family doctor or other health professional as soon as possible. You can certainly follow the advice we give, too, but your condition may need the sort of expert diagnosis and attention that a book can never give.

You may find yourself ticking boxes in more than one section because there is always a degree of overlap between the Stress Weaknesses. In this case, start with the weakness where you score the highest number of hits. When these symptoms have been successfully treated, fill in the checklists again. You will probably find that most of your problems are resolved, but if you still have problems with one or more of the other stress points, work your way through the programmes.

---

**Top tip**

When you are checking your response to the Stress Weakness Programme, you will find that most accurate assessors are other people – such as family, friends and workmates. They'll let you know exactly how you're looking and behaving.

---

### If you have not been able to pinpoint your Biotype

As you follow the Stress Weakness Programme for your most significant problem, your body will start to achieve a state of balance. As this happens, your energy levels will change and your body shape will begin to return to its natural Biotype. After four weeks, go back to Step 3 (see page 17) of the Biotype questionnaire and fill it in again. If you don't get a clear outcome, repeat on a monthly basis until you do.

## The Basic Stress Weakness Programme

This information is relevant to all Biotypes, and should be considered alongside the more specific advice for your type.

Remember, this is a gold standard. Do your best. If you come off this programme for one meal, it is not the end of the world, but it does not justify you raiding the fridge and giving up altogether for that day. Chalk it up to experience and start again. Of course, the closer you can stick to it, the quicker you will feel sparkling fit.

### You scored between 1 and 8

- Follow your Biotype diet and eat fresh seasonal food, organic wherever possible
- Avoid processed, refined or ready prepared foods
- Chew your meals well – do not try and swallow large pieces of food
- Drink plenty of still, room-temperature water – at least eight big glasses daily
- Reduce or cut out cigarettes, alcohol and caffeinated drinks; drink lots of water (see above) and weak green tea, freshly juiced fruit and vegetables, and homemade fruit spritzers
- Get plenty of rest
- Take gentle exercise in the fresh air

### You scored between 9 and 19

- Follow the above tips for lower scores
- Follow the specific supplement programme for your Stress Weakness
- Learn to relax: practise yoga or T'ai chi, swim, walk, meditate
- Have relaxing treatments, such as massage, aromatherapy, reflexology

- Assess your work stress and lighten the pressure wherever possible
- Spend your leisure time doing what you *really* enjoy. While you are treating your Stress Weakness, it's best to avoid inherently stressful activities, such as dangerous or competitive sports

**You scored over 20**
- Follow all of the advice above
- See your GP, or qualified health professional

### Supplements

To keep things simple we usually suggest taking supplements in the morning *or* in the evening (or both if you need two a day). Always take supplements with a meal. It's often easiest to put out your supplements in the morning: many health-food shops have small specially designed plastic boxes so you can carry them round with you. You may also choose to set out supplements for a week or more in separate compartments, for easy access.

You will see that several of the products listed below are by Biocare. This is because Roderick Lane has designed products for Biocare and they are his preferred product in several cases. It doesn't mean, however, that there aren't other excellent products and we have listed other quality brands and their contact details in the Directory.

### Stress weakness: Digestive function

Digestive problems are very common, but they are often simple to correct. They may exist on their own or accompany a Stress

Weakness. If you suffer from one or more of the following symptoms, follow the simple programme outlined in Chapter 4, alongside the appropriate treatment for any Stress Weakness you have.

---

### Important note

If you tick one or more of the 12 boxes in this section, you must add the total number of ticks to your score in the following sections on adrenals, thyroid, liver and hypoglycaemia.

---

### Digestive function checklist

- [ ] Frequent digestive discomfort: your stomach always/often feels uncomfortable after eating
- [ ] Temporary digestive problems; for example, mild, short-lived stomach pain (not bloating) after cheese, Chinese food, curries or other types of food
- [ ] One or more foods causes bloating, headache, nausea or increased thirst; for example, you may experience abdominal bloating after eating bread, or suffer a headache after drinking coffee
- [ ] Poor appetite
- [ ] Frequent craving for salty foods, such as crisps, salted nuts, shop-bought pizzas, etc.
- [ ] When you are tired, you crave pizza, crisps or curry (or other processed foods that are high in refined carbohydrates, fat and salt)
- [ ] Daily craving for large amounts of sugar, such as sweets, biscuits or sweet cakes, or sugared drinks
- [ ] Frequent craving for refined carbohydrates, such as

bread, pot noodles and other starch-based items including bananas

☐ Immediate craving for sweet things after eating a meal

☐ Fatigue and sleepiness immediately after eating a meal

☐ Eating relieves depression and anxiety

☐ You are often still hungry after eating a meal; however much you eat you seldom feel full or satisfied

---

## Candida and Irritable Bowel Syndrome (IBS)

Readers who have been told that they have Candida (also known as Candida albicans, yeast infection or yeast syndrome) or IBS (Irritable Bowel Syndrome) may be looking for diets specific to these two syndromes. We want to explain our approach to these two conditions, which have become catch-all explanations for problems of the digestive tract. Candida, a yeast-like bacteria that grows in the gut, has really only become a problem in the last 40 years. This is principally because of our routine exposure to antibiotics (both prescribed by the doctor and possibly also in conventionally reared livestock and the water system). Antibiotics kill the 'bad bugs' or bacteria in our digestive tract, but they also kill the good, 'healthy' ones.

The Candida yeast appears to be less sensitive to antibiotics so it is left behind. Then the lack of good bugs, means that there is no 'check' on the yeast, and it can expand to fill the available space and more.

Most of the symptoms associated with Candida overgrowth are common to all manner of digestive problems.

They are, in fact, symptoms of a generally weakened digestive tract. Our approach is to strengthen the digestive tract so that it can deal with anything nature throws at it, rather than trying to kill off Candida.

Irritable Bowel Syndrome is a name for a collection of symptoms that occur in the digestive tract. Many of these overlap with Candida and some practitioners say that it is difficult to separate the two conditions. Equally, many of the symptoms include food intolerances. You will find detailed information about dealing with digestive problems in Chapter 4.

## Stress weakness: Adrenal function

The two adrenal glands are the body's primary system for coping in times of stress. If they fail to function properly, they can cause wide-ranging effects on the body's biochemistry. The two adrenal glands sit one on top of each kidney, and produce a range of hormones, including adrenaline, the 'fight or flight' hormone that is generated so that we can respond and cope with stressful situations.

Adrenaline stimulates the liver to release stored blood sugar in order to meet the physical demands of a stress situation, such as running fast, working hard, and really focusing and concentrating on a situation.

The 'fight or flight' stress reaction evolved millions of years ago so that our ancestors could fight warring neighbours or flee from natural predators, such as the sabre-toothed tiger and mountain lion. Nowadays, however, the same power-packed explosion of chemicals is more likely to be triggered when we open bank statements, have confrontations with our

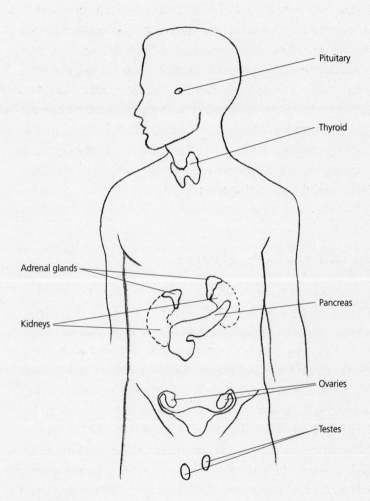

**The glands**

boss, contemplate family holidays, or sit in a traffic jam for hours.

It's not difficult to see the difference between then and now: our ancestors would have used these chemicals to fuel activity – running, hiding or fighting back, for example. In our sedentary lives today, the chemicals just swill around our bodies and pile up, potentially wreaking havoc. There is, however, one simple corrective action that can be taken to avoid this scenario. Going for a run when you have just been through a stressful experience, or simply walking fast up and down stairs, is great for calming down the situation, in order to 'use up' the adrenaline before it can cause damage. Remember, you need cardiovascular exercise (mimicking the effects of the 'fight or flight' response), not weightlifting. If the problem is long term, however, exercise on its own will not be enough. And too much exertion can actually add to the stress level, as we explain below.

If the adrenal function has become over-stressed by excessive demands, or depleted and weakened by shock and illness, the way in which it stimulates the liver can be erratic. This in turn can cause blood sugar levels to swing wildly – rather like driving a car with a rubber accelerator. Sometimes it will do what you ask; at other times the response will be completely haphazard. In the same way, if poor adrenal function is causing blood sugar to be produced erratically, you can experience weird highs and depressive lows. This is medically known as 'reactive hypoglycaemia'.

Another result of adrenal depletion can be backache. This happens because the body tries to adapt to the depletion by swelling the glands, a process called adrenal hypertrophy (literally swelling of the adrenal glands). The swollen adrenals, which have grown in much the same way as muscles that are used a lot, press on the surrounding tissue and nerves, leading to backache.

Short bursts of exercise can help suppress the pain because they trigger the release of natural painkillers called adrenal corticosteroids. But this can lead to a vicious cycle. Because the pain stops for a short time, the sufferer takes more exercise. Of course, this depletes the adrenals further, causing more problems so the sufferer tries to remedy the situation by exercising even more. Some backache sufferers exercise two or three times a day to try to relieve the discomfort caused by the underlying depletion of the adrenals. Eventually they can no longer keep up the levels of adrenal stress and stimulation to which they are subjecting their bodies to and they collapse physically, victims of the following types of conditions: chronic back pain, migraine, constant headaches, chronic fatigue, ME or glandular fever.

It doesn't end there: when you produce adrenaline you also produce a hormone called cortisol which can affect the thyroid gland and inhibit its hormone production so that it produces a poorer quality thyroxin. This results in general malaise and fatigue. You can often spot early warning symptoms such as morning fatigue, dry skin, headaches, depression, muscle aches, poor sleep, dry hair and poor skin quality.

So you can see how important it is to detect and correct any problems associated with adrenal function.

### Adrenal function checklist

Score one point for each item you tick.

**Past problems:**

☐ Were you a bedwetter as a child?

☐ Have you ever suffered temporary incontinence or bladder problems?

☐ Have you taken cortisone or any steroid medication?

☐ Have you undergone surgery under a general anaesthetic?

☐ Have you suffered from a severe debilitating illness, such as TB, hepatitis, blood poisoning, severe influenza, acute bronchial infection, asthma or any other type of serious illness?

Do you experience, or have you experienced, any of the following?

☐ Constant fatigue
☐ Insomnia
☐ Low and/or high blood pressure
☐ Pounding heart
☐ Sweating or constant cold sweats of hands and feet (often in bed)
☐ Fainting spells
☐ Migraines and severe headaches
☐ Stabbing pains behind the eyes
☐ Asthma or tight chest
☐ Neckache
☐ Backache
☐ Upper back tension, from shoulders down through top of back to shoulderblades
☐ Kidney ache (people with adrenal problems often massage the small of their back when they get up from sitting in a chair)
☐ PMS (pre-menstrual syndrome; see page 139)
☐ Clumsiness
☐ Liver spots or bronze skin patches on hands

- [ ] Alcoholic drinks go straight to your head; you're likely to be tipsy after one glass of wine
- [ ] Intolerance to cigarette smoke, perfume, exhaust fumes, cleaning fluids
- [ ] Red skin rashes or hives and skin blotches
- [ ] A dry mouth in spite of drinking plenty of water
- [ ] Desire/need to drink coffee or beverages containing caffeine every day
- [ ] Desire/need to drink alcohol every day
- [ ] Inability to tolerate hot weather or changes in temperature
- [ ] Craving for action sports, often described as being an adrenaline junkie? (if the answer is yes to this question; take a look at the thyroid checklist, page 114).
- [ ] Anxiety
- [ ] Nervousness
- [ ] Mood swings
- [ ] Poor concentration – ideas and thoughts just seemed to drift away
- [ ] Thinking about possible conflicts of any sort (rows, arguments, even discussing issues) makes you instantly tired
- [ ] You can't cope with stressful events, such as family gatherings
- [ ] You startle easily, and jump at the smallest sound
- [ ] Panic attacks
- [ ] You are easily emotional and/or have a very short fuse

### Scoring

Add up the ticks. In the ideal world, you should score zero. If that's you, go on to the rest of the Stress Weakness check-lists.

**You scored between 1 and 8**

Most adults in our stressful society will score between 1 and 8. Although this seems low, you may still feel ill. The good news, however, is that simple changes can put the problems right. Follow the Basic Stress Weakness Programme until the symptoms are no longer present.

People with adrenal stress tend to go into overdrive and ignore food so pay particular attention to eating properly. Aim for lots of fresh fruit and vegetables, lean white meat, fish and low fat dairy products. Adrenal glands respond readily to tender loving care so small changes usually have an immediate impact.

---

### Five things you can do today

1. Drink lots of still, room-temperature water and weak green tea between meals, with chamomile tea in the evening to help you relax.
2. Take a gentle walk or swim after work rather than going to the gym or playing competitive sports.
3. Have a hot shower or bath well before you go to bed: allow at least 30 minutes for your body to return to room temperature before sleep.
4. Use sweet-smelling and relaxing herbal or aromatherapeutic products in the bath/shower, such as lavender.
5. Don't watch stimulating TV programmes or films, or listen to fast or exciting music before you go to bed.

---

**Basic Stress Weakness Programme: Adrenals**

- Biotype Diet: Immediately begin to follow the diet for your Biotype. Always choose fresh produce, organic if possible.
- Reduce your intake of spices because they are stimulants and may increase anxiety symptoms.
- If you eat a lot of refined carbohydrates (such as white flour and sugar, often contained in processed foods), cut them down or, preferably, cut out completely. Look at labels and avoid foods that are sweetened with any sugars or sugar type compounds (maltose, sucrose, fructose, glucose, galactose), syrups (corn, maple or barley malt ) and sugar substitutes (including aspartame and saccharin).
- Stop adding salt to your diet, particularly if you are a Pioneer (A type).
- Assess your consumption of alcohol and cigarettes. If possible, cut them out completely. If not, ensure that you don't drink or smoke to medicate stress. If you do, you risk setting up a potentially self-destructive habit.

---

### Like water for calm

Adrenal problems are made much worse by dehydration. Carry water with you everywhere, particularly in the car and at your desk where your physical reactions to 'fight or flight' have nowhere to go except round and round your body. So before you give in to road rage or colleague fury, have a long slow drink of still water. Make sure it's at room temperature because cool or cold water will often act as a diuretic.

---

**You scored between 9 and 19**

This score represents moderate adrenal stress which, although not serious at this point, is not a positive state to be in and can spiral into an acute situation if left untreated. As well as following the suggestions for score 1 to 8, we suggest that you follow the Supplement Programme, take a serious look at your lifestyle, and re-evaluate your priorities.

*What to do*

Follow the suggestions for scores between 1 and 8 (see page 108)

Follow the supplement programme below

**Supplement programme for adrenal weakness**

Support your adrenal weakness with a programme of supplements. Take them until the problem goes away. Monitor your response by repeating the checklist monthly and noting the changes. You'll find that your most accurate assessors are other people – family, friends, workmates. They'll let you know exactly how you're doing . . .

Take:

- Biocare's vitamin B-complex in the morning
- Biocare's Beta carotene (15mg) in the morning
- Biocare's AD206, a specific herbal and nutritional product to support adrenal function *or* Core Level Adrenal by Nutri
- 2 grams of vitamin C daily, taken mid-afternoon if possible (or later in the day if you forget), preferably in the form of magnesium ascorbate or potassium ascorbate (both of which are non-acidic), rather than sodium ascorbate
- Trace mineral complex with your evening meal; try Biocare's Multi-mineral Complex or any multi-mineral

complex containing Chromium GTF (glucose tolerance factor)

- 1g magnesium with your evening meal; try Biocare Bio-magnesium or any good brand of magnesium; in combination with the trace mineral complex; this calms the mind and nerves so you sleep better

### Homeopathy

- Take 10 drops of Adrenal Liquescence complex homeopathic drops by New Vistas Ireland twice a day, about 20 minutes before breakfast and your evening meal. Take for 28 days initially; if you have improved significantly on the whole regime at that point, you can stop taking the drops. If not, take another 28-day course.

### Learn to relax

Practise your favourite forms of relaxation daily, whether they are playing music, doing yoga or T'ai chi, meditating, non-competitive swimming, gardening, cooking or walking gently in the park. Relaxation is an essential part of your life, not a luxury, so make time for it regularly every day. However busy your life is, build it into your schedule.

See Chapter 7 for our suggestions on meditation and creative visualisation.

### Assess your work stress

Reassess your work situation and the stress levels it involves and see if there are alternatives to how and/or where you work. Small changes can make a big difference:

- Make a list of everything you have to do each day (the night before, preferably, so that you can really relax when you clock off) and prioritise the items; do them in order of importance and tick them off as you complete them.

- Allow yourself more time to complete tasks: be realistic and you will find that you save yourself, and everyone else, stress and anxiety.
- Remember to add in travel and 'problem' time when you have to get from A to B.
- Always let people know if you are running late; carry a mobile phone if you are away from a land line.

---

**Top tip**

Fill the petrol tank in the car before the needle hits empty.

---

*Reconsider fun*

Consider your friends and your social life: do you move with people who are always hyped up and think that living on the edge is the only way? Parties and alcohol can be good fun and good for you – in moderation. In excess they put more pressure on your already stressed-out adrenal glands. Neither drugs or nicotine are good for you in *any* way. Make a list of all the things you really like doing, and the people you like seeing. List only the ones that give you energy, comfort and joy and build them into your life.

**You scored 20 or above**

You risk moving into the area of acute adrenal dysfunction and would be wise to address your lifestyle as well as your dietary problems immediately. Seek the advice of your GP or qualified naturopath.

If you have a history of back problems, see a chiropractor

or osteopath to check that you don't have a spinal problem, which could restrict blood supply or nerve supply and lead to the adrenals shutting down.

## Stress weakness: Thyroid function

Thyroid problems are one of the most common and widely missed hormonal dysfunctions in the Western world today. The thyroid gland regulates body metabolism through the hormone thyroxin and controls the metabolic rates of many of the cells in the body. If it is not working well, it has far-reaching effects on both your body and your brain.

People with thyroid problems, even quite slight ones, often feel that they are in some way missing out on life: they just can't quite get up enough energy to 'go for it'. The most common symptom is a constant low level fatigue. Even when they are happy and at their own physical best, people with thyroid weakness have an underlying sense of tiredness. Other common symptoms include poor digestion and weight gain, dry skin and hair, flaking finger nails, thinning frontal hair plus problems with memory, emotional stability and lack of libido.

It is possible to override a low thyroid condition by increasing adrenal stimulation through vigorous exercise. This usually reduces symptoms in the short term but it often leads to the depletion of the adrenal system as well as the thyroid. The reason for this depletion is that people feel the need to exercise hard, at least twice a day, every day, in order to maintain a sense of being 'alive'. Of course, exercise is good for you, but if you only feel alive when you are pumping iron twice a day, there is something wrong.

### Testing thyroid function

Although the main cause of thyroid dysfunction is an under-functioning thyroid gland, recent research shows that there is a secondary problem where some people under stress produce 'non-viable' thyroxin (the thyroid hormone), which is not capable of fulfilling all of its roles in the body. In other words, thyroxin is being produced in the normal way, but it is 'second grade' – rather like making paraffin when your body should be producing rocket fuel.

From a naturopathic point of view, the most accurate measurement of thyroid activity is the body's resting (or basal) temperature, which reflects your metabolic rate. This is the rate at which the body converts food and stored fats, carbo-hydrates and proteins into energy to fuel it. Your thyroid sets the metabolic rate. If thyroid function is low, so is your basal temperature and vice versa.

The best test – also the cheapest and simplest – is the Barnes Axial Temperature Test, which measures the armpit temperature, and shows the actual effect that the thyroid gland has on the cells.

### Thyroid function checklist

Score one point for each item you tick.

Do you experience, or have you experienced, any of the following?

☐ You get up feeling tired – often described as 'not being a morning person', and then your energy improves in the afternoon

☐ More sleep is not better: however long you sleep you always feel tired

- [ ] Lethargy
- [ ] Consistent low body temperature i.e., below 98.4°F (36.8°C)
- [ ] Feeling cold all the time
- [ ] Difficulty in warming up properly after getting cold
- [ ] Dry skin, tendency to eczema
- [ ] Cracking on skin of heels
- [ ] Thinning, sparse and/or brittle hair that grows slowly
- [ ] Hair loss from eyebrows
- [ ] Weak fingernails that grow slowly
- [ ] Water retention, such as puffy eyelids, swollen face, tendency to swollen feet, ankles or hands
- [ ] Cold hands and feet
- [ ] Headaches
- [ ] Migraine headaches in the front of the head or face
- [ ] Stiff joints and muscles
- [ ] Twitching in bed
- [ ] Cramps in bed
- [ ] Palpitations
- [ ] Bruise easily, sometimes for no apparent reason
- [ ] Poor digestion
- [ ] Erratic appetite and/or loss of appetite
- [ ] Weight problems or inability to lose weight
- [ ] Constipation or erratic bowel movements
- [ ] High cholesterol level
- [ ] Lack of libido
- [ ] Menstrual irregularity or difficulty
- [ ] Breast lumps
- [ ] Difficulty conceiving
- [ ] Miscarriage – inability to keep pregnancy beyond first trimester
- [ ] Greasy skin on face

☐ Slow and/or slurred speech
☐ Short-term memory loss
☐ Poor coordination, tendency to fumble
☐ Nervousness and/or nervous agitation
☐ Anxiety
☐ Seasonal Affective Disorder (SAD) – winter depression

### Scoring

Add up the ticks. As with the adrenal checklist above, you would score zero in an ideal situation. If you do, go on to the next checklist.

**You scored between 1 and 8**
Although this seems low, you may still feel unwell and tired. The good news is that simple changes to what you eat will put this right.

**Basic Stress Weakness Programme: Thyroid**
● Immediately start following the diet for your Biotype. Always choose fresh produce, organic if possible.
● If you eat a lot of carbohydrates, such as white sugars and flours and/or processed foods, cut them down or cut out.
● Avoid foods that are sweetened with sugars or sugar type compounds (maltose, sucrose, fructose, glucose, galactose), syrups (corn, maple or barley malt ) and sugar substitutes (such as aspartame and saccharin).
● Assess your consumption of alcohol and cigarettes. If possible, cut them out completely. If not, ensure that you don't drink or smoke to medicate stress. If you do, you will set up a potentially self-destructive habit.

Remember: people with thyroid weakness often eat to compensate for the sluggishness it causes so they become fridge raiders, always pecking and never sitting down to proper meals. They think they're eating like a bird when, in fact, they're consuming two to three times the calories in snacks that they would eat if they made themselves a proper meal.

---

## Five things you can do today

1. Stop drinking coffee, black tea and alcohol. Drink lots of weak green tea and still, room-temperature water.
2. Stop eating peanuts, soya in any form, cabbage (and all members of the cabbage family, such as Brussels sprouts, broccoli, kale and cauliflower) and mustard. These foods block the absorption of iodine, an essential element for the thyroid.
3. Eat shellfish for its iodine content, or deep-sea fish such as bass, haddock or cod.
4. Have an iodine rich seaweed salad, or sprinkle Nori flakes (or kelp) over your food.
5. Practise being still: stop completely for a few moments, breathe slowly and rhythmically, look out of the window into the distance.

---

**You scored between 9 and 19**

This score represents moderate thyroid stress which may escalate into an acute thyroid problem if left unchecked. Follow the Stress Weakness Programme for scores between 1 to 8 (see page 116), and also set about correcting your thyroid weakness with specially targeted nutritional supplements.

*What to do*

Follow the suggestions for scores between 1 and 8 (see page 116)

Follow the supplement programme below

---

**Top tip**

Keep warm. This will help your thyroid and give you energy. In the summer, take advantage of sunny days to get really baked. But don't forget to slap on your sunscreen. We recommend organic products, such as those produced by Green People, while the long-term safety of other products is still being evaluated. In the winter, wear warm clothes and use a sauna whenever possible to raise your core body temperature.

---

**Supplement programme for thyroid weakness**

Take these supplements until the problem goes away. Monitor your response by repeating the questionnaire monthly and noting the changes.

Take:

- One capsule of Biocare's vitamin B-complex with breakfast (beware: your urine may become very yellow, but it's perfectly healthy)
- 2 grams of vitamin C with breakfast
- 500mg L-tyrosine (an amino acid) with breakfast and your evening meal
- Trace mineral complex with your evening meal, such as Biocare's Multi-mineral Complex, or any multi mineral complex containing Chromium GTF (glucose tolerance factor)

- 500mg magnesium with your evening meal, such as Bio-care's Bio-magnesium or any good brand of magnesium; in combination with the trace mineral complex, this calms the mind and nerves so you sleep better
- Flaxseed oil, two 1 gram capsules daily, one at breakfast and one at your evening meal; you can substitute another Essential Fatty Acid (EFA) supplement, such as oil of evening primrose, borage or blackcurrant seed.

Take just one of the following:

- Kelp or seaweed (for the high iodine content): take kelp capsules, seaweed or bladderwrack capsules, or sprinkle dried seaweed flakes (called Nori or Wasabi) over food as a condiment at each meal

*or*

- TH207 by Biocare (a herbal thyroid support); take two daily, one at breakfast and one at your evening meal

*or*

- Core Level Thyro by Nutri; take two daily, one at break-fast and one at your evening meal

*Homeopathy*

Take 10 drops of Thyroid Liquescence complex homeopathic drops by New Vistas Ireland twice a day, at least 20 minutes before breakfast and your evening meal. Take for 28 days initially; if you have improved significantly on the whole regime at this stage, you can stop taking the drops. If not, take another 28-day course.

**You scored 20 or above**

You risk moving into the area of acute thyroid dysfunction and we suggest that you consult your physician or a qualified naturopath. You may need to take thyroxin, a prescription drug, for a time.

If you have a history of neck or back problems, see a chiropractor or osteopath to check that you don't have a spinal problem, which could cause restricted blood supply or nerve supply to the thyroid. This could, in turn, lead to a reduction of thyroid function. Also refer to the Spinal Function questionnaire on page 147.

## Stress weakness: Liver function

Everything that happens in your body eventually involves the liver. It's the largest and most complex organ in your body, weighing about 1.8 kilos in the average man, 1.3 kilos in women. As the central processing unit for all the daily routine functions of living – and there are more than 200 – the liver does more than any other organ or system.

### What your liver does

- Your liver is the headquarters of the bloodstream: it's the only organ with two blood supplies, one bringing newly processed nutrients from the stomach and intestines, and the other freshly oxygenated blood from the heart. Every minute, 3 pints (1.8 litres) of blood pass through it.
- The liver is also the clearing house in charge of elimination and recycling, so it is responsible for breaking down and disposing of some poisons and waste products while others are converted into beneficial compounds by liver enzymes.
- As the elimination headquarters, your liver also has a key role in your immune system (your body's defence against invaders); highly developed cells (called Kupffer cells) are

specialised rubbish collectors which destroy viruses, bacteria, dead cells, partly digested proteins in the bloodstream which can lead to allergic reactions, and any other unwanted intruders.

- The liver is the essential storage house for sugars in the form of glycogen (which give us the energy to fuel our lives), vitamins A, B and D, and trace minerals.
- The liver is intimately associated in the process of breaking down the hormones adrenaline and thyroxine and converting them into components that are used to make other beneficial chemical chains.

Your liver is extraordinarily powerful and, in a healthy state, is capable of dealing with anything that is thrown at it. The problem today is that toxic chemicals are so widespread that they accumulate, placing a continuous burden on the liver and preventing it from functioning optimally.

It is very vulnerable to damage from pollutants, the chief of which is alcohol. Routinely drinking a lot of alcohol over a long period is the primary cause of liver disease. A single alcoholic drink can potentially destroy up to one million brain cells and the same number of liver cells.

Other substances that, in excess, may cause problems for your liver include coffee, sugar, soft drinks, painkillers and other pharmaceutical drugs. This is because they increase the work the liver has to do. Because it is a synthetic hormone, the contraceptive pill also adds to the load on the liver as does HRT.

Technological pollutants such as the toner and ink in photocopiers are a problem for susceptible people, although others may be completely unaffected. The toner and ink give off solvents into the atmosphere which find their way into the liver and have to be detoxified; it's similar to the problems caused by solvent abuse, such as glue-sniffing.

### The story of the liver, the gallbladder and the importance of fat

Although they are often referred to separately, the liver and gall bladder share one function. The liver produces bile which is stored in the gall bladder, a little muscular sack which squirts out the bile into the common bile duct, where it is joined by the excreted enzymes and bicarbonates from the pancreas. The bile mixture emulsifies fats rather like a detergent. The fat becomes a cloudy, milk-like substance which the enzymes can break down. If you don't have enough bile and enzymes because of poor liver function, your body cannot break down fats. This is a big problem, because fat is essential for your body to work properly.

Good fats, also referred to as Essential Fatty Acids or EFAs (see page 127) help with a whole range of body processes from the beginning of life. Lack of sufficient EFAs may impair fertility and they are vital for the proper growth of babies in the womb, particularly for eye and brain development. If possible, prospective mothers should take EFAs for at least six months before pregnancy. Breastfeeding is important because the milk is rich in EFAs. This is believed to be one of the reasons why, in research studies, breastfed babies have a higher IQ than those who are bottlefed. (Some formula feeds now contain EFAs; look for DHA – docosahexaenoic acid – on the label.)

Good fats are good for your heart. Polyunsaturated fats (Omega-6 from plant seeds such as sunflower and soya, and Omega-3 from oily fish) are essential in your diet because your body can't make them. Omega-3 fats help to decrease pain and morning joint stiffness in rheumatoid arthritis, and may help asthmatics. Eating too few Omega-3 fats may contribute to non-insulin dependent diabetes. Monounsaturated fats (from olive or rapeseed oil, avocado and nuts) also help to lower harmful blood cholesterol and to protect against heart disease and strokes.

Recent research suggests that another essential fatty acid, eicosapentaenoic acid (EPA), may prevent weight loss in patients suffering from gastrointestinal cancer. There is also considerable research to show that EPA can help with mental disorders including all forms of depression. In fact, simply eating oily fish regularly appears to make a difference.

Another essential fatty acid called Conjugated Linolenic Acid (CLA) is brilliant for stimulating weight loss. It increases the ratio of fat burning and helps the liver's detoxification processes. CLA can be taken in supplement form, and it also occurs naturally in organic full fat milk and organic beef, the principle diet of the long, lean Masai tribe.

Eat too little fat and over time you could let yourself in for an array of symptoms, including nervous anxiety, depression and other mental disorders, restless limbs, joint stiffness, PMS, period problems, dry skin, flaking nails, dull hair, tiredness, vaginal dryness, painful intercourse and premature ageing.

## Liver function checklist

Score one point for each item you tick.

**Past problems:**

Do you have a history of any of the following?

☐ Liver conditions such as hepatitis or cirrhosis

☐ Glandular fever, Myalgic Encephalomyelitis (ME) or Epstein Barr Virus (EBV)

☐ Diabetes, either yourself or in the family

☐ Gallstones, or gall bladder removal

☐ Being persistently overweight by at least 7 or 8 pounds (about 3kg)

☐ Continual high body fat, due to being 20 pounds (about 9kg) or more overweight

☐ Working with, or consistent exposure to, dry cleaning fluids

☐ Working with, or consistent exposure to, paints, varnishes and solvents (glues)

☐ Working with, or consistent exposure to, wood preservatives or agricultural sprays and chemicals

☐ Working with, or consistent exposure to, toxic chemicals

Do you experience, or have you experienced, any of the following?

☐ Regular alcohol consumption – more than four times weekly

☐ Poor alcohol tolerance – you get tipsy or drunk very quickly

☐ Regular consumption of painkillers and/or headache or migraine preparations

☐ Poor reaction to high-sugar foods, such as increased thirst, mood swings and anxiety (see page 131)

☐ Poor reaction to chocolate, such as increased thirst, mood swings and anxiety (see page 131)

☐ Poor reaction to oily or greasy foods, such as nausea, headache, bloating and wind

☐ Natural inclination to avoid cream, butter and cheese

☐ Tendency to gain weight easily

☐ High cholesterol readings

☐ Chronic itching

☐ Migraine headaches

☐ Thick ridges on fingernails

☐ Chronic constipation

☐ Unpleasant-smelling wind

☐ Pale greasy stools that float

☐ Bleed easily, with poor blood clotting

☐ Chronic tiredness

☐ Constant desire to sleep

☐ Fatigue after eating

☐ Right-sided abdominal pain

☐ Stabbing pains under your shoulder blade/s

☐ Acute neckache

☐ 'Panda' eyes: dark circles or bags under the eyes

☐ Chemical sensitivities: do you react badly to perfume, exhaust fumes and similar environmental pollutants

### Scoring

As with adrenal and thyroid stress, you would score zero in an ideal world. But the stresses of modern life mean that many if not most people will score between 1 and 8. The good news is that simple lifestyle shifts can help.

### Five things you can do today

1. Take a few drops of Dr Bach's Rescue Remedy several times today.

2. Drink ginger tea. Either buy tea bags or, preferably, make it yourself fresh: put a grated one-inch (2.5cm) chunk of fresh peeled ginger in a pot or mug, pour on boiling water and go on topping up (the more you 'cook' the ginger, the more potent it is); you can also have this cold with ice and lemon.

3. Buy or make a fresh organic apple, carrot and ginger juice, or whiz up the flesh of a large slice of watermelon in a blender with fresh mint if you have some (see page 191).

4. Take Siberian ginseng either as a capsule or tea: put one bag in a small teapot and drink twice daily.

5. Make a big bowl of fresh organic fruit salad, with some or all of the following: apples, pears, pineapple, papaya, strawberries, blueberries, nectarines, peaches, melon, kiwi fruit and mango.

**You scored between 1 and 8**

Although this seems low, you may still feel unwell and tired. The good news is that simple changes to what you eat will put this right.

Follow the Basic Stress Weakness Programmes for Adrenal and Thyroid Weakness (see pages 109 and 116).

- The most important thing you can do to help your liver is to chew your food properly. This is explained in detail in Chapter 4. In a nutshell, eating our food slowly and chewing it thoroughly can overcome a multitude of problems because it physically reduces the biochemical load. Conversely, gobbling your food will increase the burden on an already stressed liver.

- Be sure to increase your intake of green vegetables and water.
- Decrease your consumption of coffee, tea, caffeinated drinks and sugars. Instead, drink weak green tea and plenty of still, room-temperature water.
- Get juicing! turn to Chapter 6, for details of our 5-Day Juice Detox Programme.
- If you regularly eat saturated fats (see page 128) cut down as much as possible, and be careful about how much unsaturated oil and fat you eat. Monitor how you feel when you eat any sorts of fats and oils; if they make you feel nauseous or bring a recurrence of the symptoms, try to eat as little as possible until you feel better. Do not, however, forget that fats perform vital functions in our bodies and a total non-fat diet is dangerous for longer than a few weeks.

---

**Fat facts**

**Unsaturated 'good' fats**

Eat lots of the following, which contain essential fatty acids (EFAs; also known as omega 3 and 6 oils):

- Oily fish, such as mackerel, herrings, kippers, pilchards, trout, salmon, sardines, fresh tuna and anchovies
- Full fat organic milk
- Vegetables, such as sweet potatoes, peanuts, green leafy vegetables
- Avocados

---

- Nuts, seeds walnuts, almonds and linseeds (ground)
- Olive, rapeseed, soya and sunflower oils
- EFA supplements, including evening primrose oil, starflower (borage) and blackcurrant seed oil, linseed oil, flaxseed oil, hemp oil

### Saturated 'bad' fats

Eat in moderation:

- Meat, such as organic beef, chicken, venison and lamb
- Eggs

Both meat and eggs are considered to be 'bad fats' because they are saturated; however, they contain usable fats for the body and can be healthy, provided you choose lean cuts and eat them in moderation. Always grill meats if possible, which preserves their EFA content. Always choose organic. Organic beef, like full-fat organic milk, contains EFA, while non-organic does not. Remember to trim all surplus fat before cooking.

Cut down on:

- Lard
- Dripping
- Coconut oil
- Palm oil
- Conventionally produced margarine – this has no nutritional value and, although it is neither a good nor a bad fat, your liver/gall bladder still has to deal with it
- Butter and hard cheese – cut down on these if they do not suit your Biotype

**You scored between 9 and 19**

This score suggests a modest level of liver stress which, although not currently serious, may be making you feel physically and mentally low. It may spiral into an acute problem if left untreated.

We suggest you follow the suggestions for score 1 to 8 and the Liver Function Support Programme. Additionally, because people with poor liver function tend to get angry quickly ('feeling liverish'), it's important to nurture all aspects of your life. Any stress-induced hormonal swing, bilious attack, headache or over-exertion of any kind will give the liver more work instead of letting it heal. So get plenty of rest, take gentle exercise in the fresh air and spend some of your time doing things you like with friends.

*What to do*

Follow the suggestions for scores between 1 and 8 (see page 126)

Follow the liver function support programme below.

**Liver function support programme**

The emphasis here is on cleansing and supporting the liver. Take:

- 2 grams of vitamin C, one with breakfast and one with lunch (choose the non-acidic formations, such as potassium ascorbate or magnesium ascorbate)
- 50mg vitamin B3 (niacin), once a day with breakfast

Comforting teas:

- Ginger tea: buy tea bags or make fresh ginger tea. Peel and grate a one-inch (2.5cm) lump of root ginger, pour boiling water over it and leave for five or, preferably, 10 minutes. Drink whenever your digestion needs calming.

If you don't like ginger, try one of the following. The general instructions are the same for each one: pour boiling water over the herb, leave to infuse for five or 10 minutes, sieve if you wish, then drink.

- Liquorice root tea: grind the root into a coarse powder and add two heaped teaspoons (10ml) to a mug of boiling water. Drink three times daily
- Fenugreek seed tea: one teaspoon (5ml) to a mug of boiling water; drink three times daily.
- Dandelion root tea: one heaped teaspoon (5ml) to a mug of boiling water; drink three times daily.

You should see a significant improvement from the supplements and the ginger (or other) tea in tandem with following your Biotype diet. If, after 28 days, you are not feeling significantly better, add in one of the following:

- Biocare's Hepaclear-T (liver support tea), 5 mugs daily, prepared as directed on the packet

*or*

- Swedish Bitters (a blend of herbs for liver function, available from healthfood shops), three times daily between meals

*or*

- Core Level Liver by Nutri; take twice daily at breakfast and your evening meal

*or*

- Biocare's Hep 194; take twice daily with food
- You could also try taking 1000mg capsule of the herb milk thistle; take daily for four weeks.

*Homeopathy*

Take one teaspoonful of Liver Liquescence complex homeo-pathic drops by New Vistas Ireland three times daily, between meals. Take for 28 days initially; if you have improved significantly on the whole regime at this stage, you can stop taking the drops. If not, take another 28-day course.

**You scored 20 or over**

You risk moving into a state of potential liver crisis and should consult your GP or other qualified health professional immediately. The liver is the key player in all physiological functions; if you have any continuous liver problems you should seek qualified help immediately. The liver is a very resilient organ, but that has an in-built drawback. Because of its outstanding ability to repair itself, people suffering from liver disorders can struggle along for years unaware of a potentially serious problem such as gallstones or a low level hepatic infection.

## Stress weakness: Sugar-processing problems – hypoglycaemia

Hypoglycaemia means 'low blood sugar', and is characterised by fluctuating blood sugar levels. It is not a disease but a symptom indicating that the body's system, which controls the processing of sugars (and this includes the thyroid, adrenals, pituitary, liver and pancreas), has become erratic. It happens if the input of glucose (the sugar energy base) into the bloodstream is not enough to keep pace with the rate at which it is being used. In a nutshell, more glucose is going out than coming in.

The first description of this condition occurred in the Book of Genesis. After working in the fields, Esau felt so faint that he was sure he was going to die. His brother Jacob agreed to give him a bowl of red lentil soup in return for his birthright. In fact, Esau was so revived by the pottage that he was able to carry on as usual (minus his birthright . . .).

The most common cause of 'modern' hypoglycaemia is eating too many refined processed foods, particularly white sugar and white flour. This is because they lack the full spectrum of natural nutrients. Without these vitamins, minerals and trace elements, the sugar-regulating machinery can't work properly. Eating refined foods occasionally is unlikely to cause a problem, but case histories of hypoglycaemics invariably show that their diets centre round processed foods and lots of refined sugar.

A balanced blood sugar level is essential for the brain and central nervous system – which together govern the way we think and behave – to operate efficiently. At its most severe, hypoglycaemia can turn intelligent, calm, collected people into stuttering, shaking wrecks who find it hard to get their lives together – look at Esau. Our brains and nervous systems also control our hormones so low blood sugar affects them, too. Because blood sugar influences the liver, adrenals and thyroid, hypoglycaemia plays a part in a wide range of conditions including:

- asthma
- hay fever
- eczema
- sinus problems
- rheumatoid arthritis
- acute rheumatic fever and other allergy-related, inflammatory conditions
- diabetes mellitus

- multiple sclerosis (MS)
- peptic ulcer
- heart disease
- Meniere's syndrome (a disorder of the inner ear, which includes vertigo, ringing in the ears, and fluctuating hearing loss)
- fatigue and exhaustion
- neuropsychiatric disorders, such as depression, hypermania, schizophrenia, nervous breakdown, alcoholism, addiction and anorexia
- antisocial behaviour including hyperactivity and delinquency
- under-achievement in children
- PMS (pre-menstrual syndrome) and menstrual irregularity

Because the nervous system (brain and spinal chord) is so dependent on a continuous adequate supply of glucose to work normally, the most obvious and dramatic symptoms of hypoglycaemia are usually neurological and psychiatric. Hypoglycaemic episodes can mimic almost every neurological and psychiatric disorder so it is vital to have a correct diagnosis before patients are given inappropriate drugs or other treatment.

If blood sugar levels fall quickly below normal, adrenaline is released and the following symptoms, which resemble a panic attack, are likely:

- sweating
- night sweats
- weakness
- hunger
- rapid beating of the heart
- feeling of fear or anxiety

If blood sugar levels drop slowly over two hours or more, the symptoms include:

- headache
- blurred vision
- mental confusion
- double vision
- incoherent speech
- coma (rare)
- convulsions (also rare)

If hypoglycaemia persists over a period of hours, a number of possible symptoms result:

- outbursts of temper
- extreme depression
- prolonged sleepiness
- restlessness
- negativism
- personality changes
- emotional instability
- maniacal behaviour

### Low blood sugar (hypoglycaemia) checklist

Score one point for each item you tick.

Have you ever had any or all of the following results from medical tests or examinations:

☐ Diagnosis of diabetes
☐ Diagnosis of low blood sugar (hypoglycaemia)
☐ Has sugar ever been found in your urine
☐ Have ketones ever been found in your urine

Do you experience, or have you experienced, any of the following?

- ☐ Your urine smells of pear drops
- ☐ You are constantly thirsty
- ☐ You have itchy ears
- ☐ You constantly need to urinate
- ☐ You always want to eat when you're nervous
- ☐ You have an excessive appetite (you might buy five doughnuts for workmates, eat them all yourself, and have to go back to buy another five)
- ☐ You are constantly hungry between meals
- ☐ You become irritable before meals
- ☐ Meals are a time of conflict in your family
- ☐ You tremble or get shaky between meals, not necessarily when you're hungry
- ☐ You become faint if you miss or delay a meal
- ☐ Your heart pounds or palpitates if you miss a meal
- ☐ Eating relieves symptoms, such as fatigue and shaking
- ☐ You get tired after eating
- ☐ You wake up with a headache
- ☐ You get afternoon headaches
- ☐ Eating sweets, cakes and biscuits makes you feel nauseous
- ☐ You crave coffee, tea or sweet snacks in the afternoon
- ☐ You regularly have mood swings or unaccountable moments of anguish and depression
- ☐ You have an abnormal or constant desire to eat sweets or snacks
- ☐ You have no desire to eat at all
- ☐ You have developed a recent food craving
- ☐ You have a craving for lots of bananas or carrots
- ☐ You wake up in the early hours of the morning needing a snack

☐   Cuts and bruises heal slowly

☐   You're constantly prey to viruses and small infections

## Scoring

As with the other stress points, you would ideally score none. If this is the case, carry on.

### You scored between 1 and 8

This score is very common for many adults today. Although this does not indicate a serious problem, you may still feel low and your energy and state of health are probably not consistently at their best. Simple changes can put this problem right. The key is to balance your sugar levels through your daily diet by taking the strain off your pancreas, liver and adrenals. Follow this eating plan and do not cheat if you want it to work!

### Basic Stress Weakness Programme: hypoglycaemia

This diet programme consists of three moderate meals plus between-meal snacks and a snack before bedtime. The golden rules are:

- Meals must be on time without exception; choose your own times but never go more than three hours without a meal or a snack
- Snacks such as nuts, seeds, rice cakes, Ryvita, trail mix (without raisins) are essential to provide a level intake of nutrients
- Eat absolutely no refined foods (sugar or other processed products)
- Don't drink any caffeine-containing drinks

Do eat:

- All meat, poultry, fish and seafood
- All dairy products (eggs, milk, butter, cheese, yoghurt)
- Nuts
- Old-fashioned nut butters, such as peanut, cashew and almond (choose brands without any added sugar or honey)
- Whole-grains (brown rice, whole-wheat, whole-rye, oats, spelt, farro, kamut)

Don't eat:

- Any sugars, including honey and molasses
- White flour products, such as noodles, pasta or white rice
- Dates, raisins or other dried fruit ( too high in sugar content)
- Any soft drinks and fruit juices that have additives such as sugar of any kind, preservatives or flavourings. They may be marked 'freshly squeezed', but check the label
- Coffee or strong tea
- Pies, cakes, pastries, confectionery, ice-cream
- Any alcoholic beverages

*Snacks are vital*

Make sure you eat snacks between meals so that your blood sugar is fuelled every three hours. Choose snacks from the 'eat lots of' section of your Biotype diet.

Wise choices are:

- Nuts and seeds
- Full-fat milk shakes; you can add fresh fruit but no sugar
- Fresh hard fruit, such as apples or pears
- Ryvita and oatcakes
- In the case of hypoglycaemia, fats can be beneficial, so a

good snack would be an oatcake or Ryvita with organic butter and 1oz (25g) cheese
- If you can't find anything else, it's better to have a processed cheese slice or the meat part of a burger than go hungry

**You scored between 9 and 19**
This score represents moderate hypoglycaemia. Hypoglycaemia can affect all hormone functions, so although your condition is not severe at the moment it may spiral into an acute problem if left untreated.

Follow the Stress Weakness Programme for scores between 1 to 8 (see page 136), and also set about correcting your thyroid weakness with specially targeted nutritional supplements.

*What to do*
- Follow the suggestions for scores between 1 and 8 (see page 136)
- Follow the supplement programme below
- If you are also treating another Stress Weakness, do not duplicate supplements

**Supplement programme for hypoglycaemia**
Take:

- Vitamin B-complex, one capsule in the morning
- Chromium GTF, 200 mcg with breakfast
- Digestive enzymes with each meal. Try to get Polyzyme Forte by Biocare, if possible; if you have a definite sensitivity reaction to a specific food group, such as bloating with wheat, or a headache after coffee, take Spectrumzyme by Biocare
- Sucroguard by Biocare, twice daily at breakfast and your

evening meal or Carbomet by Nutri, one with each meal
- Multi-Mineral Complex by Biocare, one with your evening meal
- Magnesium (500mg) with evening meal; choose Biocare Bio-magnesium or any good brand of magnesium; in combination with the trace mineral complex, this calms the mind and nerves so you sleep better

**You scored 20 or over**
You are moving into a state of possible hypoglycaemia crisis and should consult your GP or other qualified health professional immediately. Blood sugar disorders can cause potentially serious problems such as falling asleep while driving, migraine, visual disturbances, inability to focus, anxiety and panic attacks.

---

### Blood sugar and PMS (pre-menstrual syndrome)

At least half of women who are menstruating suffer from some sort of problem in the 10 days or so leading up to their period. There are about 150 symptoms associated with this problem. Some of the most common are:

- feeling bloated
- weight gain
- discomfort in breasts, back or lower abdomen
- irritability
- depression
- aggression
- anxiety and tension
- tiredness
- loss of concentration

---

PMS (pre-menstrual syndrome) is a group of some 150 symptoms, which affect health on all levels, including emotional well-being. The term PMT (pre-menstrual tension) was once widely used for the psychiatric or emotional symptoms leading up to a period, but PMS is now used to cover all of the wide variety of symptoms that can appear. True PMS affects between 3 and 8 per cent of women. The most severe form of PMS is called pre-menstrual dysphoric disorder (PMDD), in which the emotional symptoms such as depression, mood swings, anxiety and tension are significantly worse.

The most commonly accepted definition of this hormonal illness is 'the recurrence of symptoms in the "premenstruum" with the absence of symptoms in the "postmenstruum".' This definition means that:

1. The symptoms occur exclusively in the second part of the menstrual cycle (known as the luteal phase)
2. There is a complete absence of symptoms after the onset of the heaviest day of menstruation for at least seven days
3. Symptoms recur during three successive cycles

By using this definition, PMS is not confused with chronic illnesses, because of the complete absence of symptoms during menstruation.

Some health practitioners believe that the only effective method of managing PMS is synthetic progesterone therapy; in practice, this is not always the case. A large number of sufferers achieve no significant benefit from progesterone therapy; only 29 per cent of women in one major study experienced just 50 percent relief of symptoms, and in other cases there was initial improvement, which subsequently faded.

In the last five or so years, Prozac and other mood-altering pharmaceutical drugs, such as the benzodiazepine (Xanax), have also been prescribed for PMS. However, as with all drugs, Prozac and Xanax have side-effects, which often get worse with higher doses. A multi-centre trial showed that women with PMS had significantly lower levels of tensions, irritability and dysphoria when taking these drugs. But the group taking 60 mg Prozac daily reported a high level of side-effects.

Common side effects of Prozac include:

- Gastro-intestinal disorders, including nausea, vomiting, dyspepsia, diarrhoea, constipation and abdominal pain
- Hypersensitivity reactions
- Dry mouth
- Nervousness
- Anxiety
- Headache
- Insomnia
- Loss of libido and sexual dysfunction

Common side effects of Xanax, which in one trial helped 37 per cent of women, particularly with irritability and sadness, include:

- Drowsiness
- Sedation
- Blurring of vision
- Unsteadiness

More rarely, adverse effects of Xanax may include:

- Concentration difficulties
- Confusion

- Hallucinations
- Stimulation, irritation, agitation, rage, aggression and hostile behaviour

Like many hormonal problems, more than one system is involved in PMS. As well as erratic oestrogen and progesterone levels, adrenaline and thyroxine are implicated. Look back at the thyroid and adrenal checklists and you will find all of the most common PMS symptoms.

The solution is to treat blood sugar regulation, the factor that is common to all three hormonal regulatory systems (adrenals, thyroid and the reproductive system) and the liver. Balancing your blood sugar will greatly reduce mood swings; most sufferers also find that the cramping improves and that the length of periods is reduced as well.

## What to do

If you suffer PMS, think of your hormonal system as the central heating in a house. The glucose carrying blood is like the circulating hot water, the hormones are the time clock and the adrenal response influenced by your blood sugar levels is the thermostat. The problem with your hormonal central heating is that the control mechanism works erratically, due to the problems we have talked about above (in other words, problems with adrenals, thyroid, reproductive system and liver function). This causes sudden drops in blood sugar, and these dips and surges trigger mood swings ranging from tearfulness to homicidal rage.

The temptation then is to stuff chocolate biscuits in your mouth, which may make you feel better temporarily but is in fact making the problem worse. The most effective way to put your control mechanism right is to keep your blood sugar steady and balanced by eating at regular three-hourly intervals. Putting the food in your mouth is rather like manually switching on the system to heat up the water, so that the house never gets cold.

Even if you aren't hungry, you must eat at three-hourly intervals. The desire not to eat can be, in some instances, an indicator of a drop in blood sugar, which will, in turn, lead to an adrenaline 'burst', with the rash of symptoms linked to that (see page 105). Follow the recommendations for hypoglycaemia, and be certain to eat snacks between meals (see page 136).

Eating in this way doesn't imply an invitation to overeat. You should be eating moderate amounts at regular intervals. Under no circumstances should you miss or delay a snack or meal; the same applies to any nutritional products that you may have been advised to take. For some women with a severe PMS-management problem, missing or delaying a meal or snack by 15 minutes can bring on a hypoglycaemic attack, which can lead to several days of misery. You may need to exert a lot of self-control in the two weeks before your period, and during it. But the results will be worth it.

As all hormones are processed via the liver, good liver function is also crucial to the entire process. So fill in the Liver Function checklist (see page 124) and follow the appropriate advice for your score in the Liver Stress Weakness Programme. As before, please don't duplicate supplements.

## Spinal stress

### Spinal function

Most people never give a thought to their spines. Yet your entire body's muscular, nervous, organ and glandular network is either hanging from or balanced on your spine. Your spinal chord is the information superhighway between your brain and your body via your nervous system. It affects your thoughts, memory, learning and your whole consciousness, or awareness of life. So it needs to be in good shape.

Many people think that you should only visit an osteopath or chiropractor if your back is painful. In fact, spinal problems very often refer down an arm or leg. So the central focus of a spinal problem will become a major joint, such as the hip, knee or elbow.

Some spinal problems do not actually cause pain and only manifest by causing general weakness, such as a weak arm or a leg that is hard to lift when walking up a staircase. Sometimes, because of referred pain, the spinal problem will 'refer' (travel to a different but connected part of the body) and mimic the sensation of arthritis, tingling, weakness or pain in a joint or muscle (see illustration on page 145).

This is all well known theory, and may be picked up by conventional medical tests. What often slips through the conventional net, however, is the problem of distorted neural feedback to the internal organs. This may sound complicated, but it's really quite straightforward. It works like this: when a nerve is slightly compressed, it can react a bit like a garden hose with a kink in it – the tap is full on but only a trickle comes out. The desperate organ or gland demands more and more and gets less and less until finally it is exhausted and stops working.

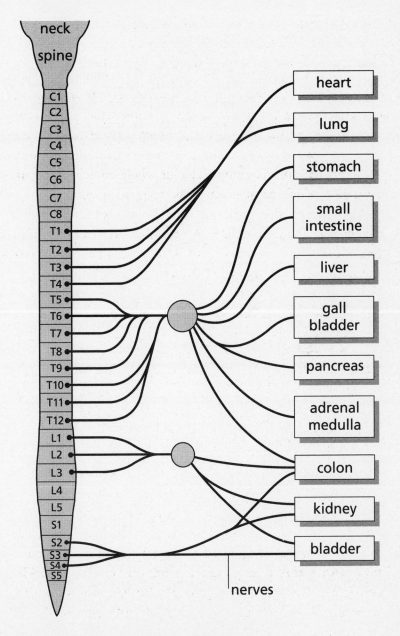

The spine and its relationship to glands and organs

Being overweight can be a significant factor in this: the more weight you carry, the more tendency to nerve compression. Carrying 10 to 20 pounds (4 to 9kg) of excess weight is the equivalent of carrying a small child – or a rucksack containing 20 cans of beans – around all day, then sleeping with the child (or the beans) on your chest all night.

Having a bad back can make your life miserable. Not only is it painful in its own right, but a spinal problem can influence an incredibly wide range of physical and emotional functions through the nervous system. Nerves control blood vessels, glandular function, pain, touch and sensation. In fact they deliver all of your experiences, both internal and external. A damaged spine can even affect your immune system, which means that infections take longer to clear up.

Although a spinal problem is remarkably easy to acquire and virtually all of us will have had one at some point, most spinal problems are self-balancing and rectifying. They usually occur after some form of physical trauma such as lifting, car accidents, repetitive movements (such as typing), bad sleeping habits (like sleeping on several pillows and a soggy mattress), even poorly designed sofas and car seats, all of which contribute to a subtle adaptation and distortion of the spine. Once the spine goes out of correct alignment, it can irritate, compress and sometimes pinch the delicate nerves. This, as we described in the sections on Thyroid and Adrenal Weakness (pages 113 and 102), can affect the functioning of glands and organs.

Treating a spinal problem can take a short or long time. In general, the longer you have had the problem, the more treatment you need. It is well worthwhile addressing spinal and dietary problems together.

## Spinal function checklist

Score one point for each item you tick.

Have you ever had any or all of the following results from medical tests or examinations:

☐ High or low blood pressure

☐ Swollen liver (this causes internal displacement, which puts pressure on the spine and spinal nerves) or hepatic migraine

Do you experience, or have you experienced, any of the following?

☐ Headaches

☐ Fatigue

☐ Erratic vision

☐ Hearing problems such as tinnitus or directional deafness (in other words, partial hearing)

☐ Sinus headache – feels like a migraine at the front of your head

☐ Aching sinuses – may come from pressure on nerves and/or discs in the neck

☐ Sinus pressure – feels like your sinuses have been pushed in or punched

☐ Hay fever or other allergies to air-borne particles that irritate the sinus passage, such as diesel/car fumes, pollens, household dust, tobacco smoke, dust mites or fine sawdust

☐ Sore throat

☐ Cough

☐ Tonsillitis

☐ Hoarseness and fading voice

☐ Shortness of breath

- [ ] Stiff neck
- [ ] Pain in shoulders
- [ ] Pain in the neck, or running up the side of it
- [ ] Tennis elbow
- [ ] Chest pains
- [ ] Tight chest
- [ ] Muscle aches
- [ ] Muscular stiffness
- [ ] Joint aches
- [ ] Sciatica
- [ ] Knee ache/pains
- [ ] Lower back pain
- [ ] Pain at the end of spine
- [ ] Weak legs
- [ ] Erratic menstrual cycle
- [ ] PMS
- [ ] Adrenal stress symptoms
- [ ] Thyroid stress symptoms
- [ ] Blood sugar irregularities
- [ ] Kidney pains
- [ ] Indigestion
- [ ] Irritable bowel syndrome (IBS)
- [ ] Constipation
- [ ] Bladder irritation
- [ ] Prostate problems
- [ ] Haemorrhoids

### Scoring

**You scored between 1 and 8**

Research shows that by far the majority of adults have suffered back pain at some point. While it's not a serious problem, it can still account for your feeling incredibly low. Simple stretching and postural exercises (see page 150), plus drinking lots of water and relaxing, will often rectify a low score such as this.

---

**Top tip**

Never sleep with more than one pillow; try an orthopaedic pillow or a soft feather one which you can bunch up to support your neck.

---

**You scored between 9 and 19**

This represents a moderate degree of spinal misalignment. If left unchecked, it may quickly spiral into an acute problem. If you find yourself in this area we suggest you look closely at your posture and your seating arrangements at work, home and in the car. A soggy mattress can also contribute to the problem: if buying a new firm one is impossible, try putting a board under your mattress. If you have a consistently aching back after driving, try using a lumbar roll (available from the Back Shop). Again, if watching TV sends you in spinal ache or spasm, make sure that you are sitting upright (see page 152) and that the screen is straight ahead of you; also practise stretches (see page 150) while you are watching.

If you belong to a gym you would be well advised to avoid lifting weights until you have a stable spinal and muscular skeletal system. Movement systems such as yoga, T'ai chi, Feldenkrais, Pilates and ballet can be very helpful (see page 273 for details). Hands-on therapies such as the Alexander Technique (which you can also do on your own), Hellerwork, Rolfing and muscle-based physiotherapy are very useful.

Any high score on the Spinal Function checklist should be taken quite seriously and you may want to consider consulting a registered chiropractor or osteopath at this point.

**You scored 20 or over**
You are moving into the area of acute spinal dysfunction and may well need specialist treatment for a time. We suggest you consult a chiropractor or osteopath, or a qualified naturopath, as well as following the advice above.

## Stretches

Do these stretches at least once a day and preferably more often. You can do several of these stretches sitting down – so they're great for desk work, watching TV or travelling, as well as for anyone who is unable to stand for any reason. Hold each stretch for 10 seconds then build up to 60 seconds. Remember to keep breathing slowly and rhythmically – don't hold your breath. If any position is painful, stop immediately and see your health professional if the pain continues.

- Full-body stretch 1: Stand on your tip toes and reach your fingertips up to the heavens so that your spine lengthens.
- Full-body stretch 2: Sitting or lying down, point your toes away from your body and stretch your fingers above your head, as far as both will go.
- Full-body stretch 3: Stand with your feet aligned with your hips, arms hanging gently at your sides and sway slowly from side to side; as you rock to the left, tilt your head to the right and vice versa; let your right

heel come up as you sway to the left, your left as you go to the right. Do this with a slow rhythmic motion, and hum a lullaby or traditional Black spiritual at the same time.

- Back stretch: Sitting or standing, align your feet with your hips, lift your arms forward and up to shoulder level, interlock your fingers and press them away from you, palms facing you; keep your chin dropped.
- Chest stretch: Sitting or standing, bring your hands behind your back at bum height; interlock your fingers with the palms up, then push your hands down and out behind you as far as is comfortable.
- Seated stretch: sit on the floor, legs apart, then slowly walk your hands forward, fingers spread; when you have gone as far as you can, hold for 10 to 60 seconds before walking them back.
- Groin stretch: sit on the floor, knees apart, and bring the soles of your feet together.

## Walk tall

Your posture paints a pretty accurate picture of how you feel. When you are depressed, you look low – hunched over and peering at the ground. You can help your spine, and your mood, by standing tall and looking ahead of you. Imagine a gold thread running from the crown of your head up into the sky. Feel positive – and look it.

## Sitting at the computer or TV

Many spinal problems are due to the way we distort our bodies at our desks and at computer screens. These simple guidelines will help your posture:

- Keep your feet placed flat on the floor; adjust the height of your chair seat if necessary
- Your seat should support your back so that it is straight but not pushed forward
- The edge of your chair should not press into the back of your knees or cause pressure on the backs of your thighs
- Do not slouch in front of the screen; sit on the front part of your sitting bones and keep your head upright
- If you are working at a VDU screen or looking at a TV, it should be elevated so that the top is directly in front of your eyes rather than down
- The screen should be directly in front of you so that you do not twist your spine to work at it
- If you tense up sitting at your desk, hum in a low key from your chest – this vibrates the chest cavity and relaxes the internal musculature

# 4

# Digestion, Food Intolerances and the Chew, Chew Cult

Food intolerances (also called allergies or sensitivities) have become the villain of the late 20th century, blamed for a rag bag of common problems from bloating, wind and nausea to fatigue after eating, headache, constipation, diarrhoea, water retention around the abdomen and, of course, abdominal weight gain.

These symptoms also cross over into those linked with irritable bowel syndrome (IBS) and Candida (also called yeast infection or yeast syndrome). Many practitioners admit that it is difficult to separate out the various conditions and establish a definite cause. However, as we said in the last chapter, we believe that the main villain underlying all these is an unhealthy digestive tract.

The problems usually start when we first put food in our mouths – in other words, with chewing (or the lack of it), which leads to a chain of disasters in our digestive tract. We have explained this more fully below but, in brief, the more you chew, the smaller the particles that reach the stomach and the easier they are to digest. Chewing also stimulates the production of hydrochloric acid (stomach acid), digestive enzymes and bile, which allow foods to be processed properly.

Having said that, there is no doubt that some people are

intolerant of some foods, but following the diet for your Biotype should guide you to foods that suit you and your constitution. By chewing meals properly and eating the foods that suit their Biotype, as well as identifying and correcting any Stress Weaknesses, many people find that the problems disappear altogether.

---

**Warning**

True (also known as 'classical') allergies that affect the immune system can be very dangerous, indeed potentially fatal. The most common food causes of these are peanuts, fish, shellfish and wheat (as in coeliac disease). If you are concerned that you may suffer from a true allergy, you should consult your family doctor and follow conventional medical advice at all times. See the Directory (see page 278) for details of how to contact the Anaphylaxis Campaign.

---

## How do you find out what food is bothering your body?

Start by following your individual Biotype diet. Then identify and treat any Stress Weaknesses.

If you still have problems after four weeks, work your way through this stage-by-stage programme to help find the cause of your symptoms, and then correct it.

### Step 1
### Likely problem: weak digestion

Solution:
- Chew your food properly; work it in your mouth until you

can feel that it is in very small pieces, then swallow. If the food is starchy, swallow when it turns sweet.

- Don't eat on the run and don't leap up from the table until you have finished your food properly.
- If possible, sit for 10 minutes after you have finished eating. Take a gentle walk after dinner.

If that makes only a marginal difference to your symptoms, or no difference at all, go on to Step 2.

## Step 2
### Likely problem: deficiency of digestive enzymes

Solution:

- If the problem seems to occur only when you eat meat, take digestive enzymes (such as Polyzyme forte by Biocare) and hydrochloric acid supplements (such as Hypo-D by Nutri or HCL and Pepsin by Biocare) with each meal. Do not take HCL supplements if you have an ulcer.
- If you have problems with foods other than meat, take digestive enzyme supplements with each meal

  If that makes no difference, go on to Step 3.

## Step 3
### Likely problem: a true food intolerance

Solution:

- Seek qualified help from your GP, a physician with a special interest in food intolerance (there are few of these so you may have to be determined) or a naturopath or appropriately qualified nutritionist. See the Directory (page 273) for more information and contacts.

## Your digestion: the real story

### The chew, chew cult

The most common cause of digestive problems and food sensitivities is not chewing our food. Not enough, and often not at all. This gives rise to a whole chain of events which mean that our digestion doesn't work properly, can't deal with food and makes us ill.

Now compare what *should* happen when we eat, with what usually goes on.

### The digestive process: what *should* happen

*Stage 1: mind and body*

- Good digestion starts in the mind when we feel hungry and start to prepare food.
- Our senses get into a happy state of anticipation: think of what happens when you smell coffee brewing, bread baking or the scent of ripe peaches. Or when you wander round a market looking at the colours and textures of fresh seasonal food. Your mouth literally waters.
- Saliva is crucial to the digestive process because it causes the release of a digestive enzyme calls 'ptyalin'. This tells your brain that sustenance is on the way and your brain sends the message to your digestive system to fire up.
- When you chew your food, the starch content begins to dissolve in your mouth and converts into sugars. These pre-digested sugars reinforce the message to the brain.
- But chewing does far more than that. It prepares your

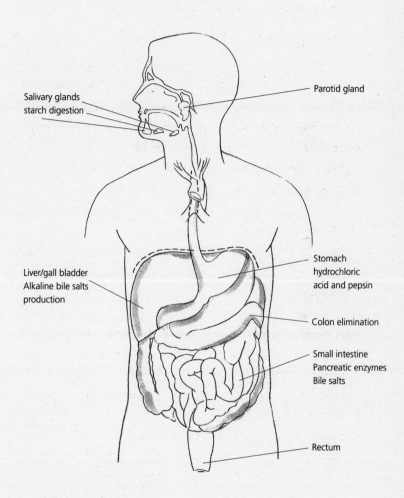

Parotid gland

Salivary glands
starch digestion

Stomach
hydrochloric
acid and pepsin

Liver/gall bladder
Alkaline bile salts
production

Colon elimination

Small intestine
Pancreatic enzymes
Bile salts

Rectum

**The digestive tract**

food to be digested and the nutrients absorbed into your body – the point of the exercise.

*Stage 2: the stomach*
- As the small masticated pieces of food pass into your stomach, hydrochloric acid is formed, which dissolves the chewed food so that it can be used by the body. Rather like a washing machine, the stomach tumbles the food and acid round and round, turning the masticated mass into a soupy liquid.

*Stage 3: the duodenum (small intestine)*
- The food/acid soup meets the alkaline bile and enzyme mix that is produced by the pancreas, liver and gallbladder. This stage is vitally important because it is here that the nutrients are absorbed into the bloodstream.

**The digestive process: what *usually* happens**

*Stage 1*
- We feel hungry, grab a sandwich, chocolate bar or packet of crisps and stuff it in our mouths, not even bothering to sit down. If we're at home, we raid the fridge or larder.
- We don't chew this food so the digestive enzyme ptyalin is not produced in adequate quantities. The brain isn't prepared for food and neither is the digestive system. It's a case of assault and battery.
- Gulping and bolting our food means that we take in with it large quantities of air, which most probably leads to excessive wind. Sometimes this is so severe that it causes stomach cramps and bloating, plus

heartburn and acid reflux, which pushes up through our digestive tract and causes a bitter taste in the mouth.

---

**Top tip**

Soothe heartburn by sucking peppermints, drinking peppermint tea or taking a small spoonful of oil of peppermint (sold as Colpermin).

---

*Stage 2: the stomach*

- Because we haven't chewed our food properly, the stomach has to produce lots of hydrochloric acid to dissolve the large resistant food particles. The combination of gulping air (see above) plus the extra acid often results in acid belches.

- You are likely to eat more than you need because your brain has not registered that you are eating.

*Stage 3: the duodenum (small intestine)*

- Remember this area is where acid meets alkaline: every schoolchild knows that this mixture has the potential to produce heat and liberated gas. So pushing the delicate balance out of kilter can easily produce undesirable side-effects.

- There are several potential trouble spots. If your stomach has had to produce lots of acid to dissolve the unchewed food or if you have eaten acid-forming foods (such as vinegar, citrus fruits, acid wine or champagne) it is possible to swamp and push out the essential alkaline materials.

- Very spicy foods also cause a problem because they can irritate the digestive tract and, in some cases, cause inflammation. Sugary foods are a hazard, too, because they trick the brain into thinking that the digestive process is over. This is because the brain believes that sugar is only a small percentage of the food we are eating. The brain registers sugar at two points of the digestive process. Firstly, at the point of chewing – if you chew your food properly you will break it down and the sugar signal will go to your brain. Secondly, at the point after carbohydrates have been assimilated into the bloodstream from the small intestine. If a lot of sugar hits the brain, it doesn't register that it came from the mouth rather than the small intestine, it simply reckons that the small intestine must be full and so digestion must be complete. Of course, this isn't the case: when the brain gets the sugar hit, the intestine may be full of undigested or partially digested food. The brain is working on false information, which occurs because refined sugars are absorbed more or less instantly. That's why they can almost immediately lift a diabetic from a coma.

### Look after your mouth

The mouth is critical to the digestion because it is designed to safeguard the body from unwanted substances, acting both as a screening system and filter. Bad gums, tooth decay, poor-quality fillings all slowly leak contaminants into the digestive tract. Gums and teeth that are in bad condition are often one of the basic causes of poor digestion. So poor gums and teeth will often act as an indicator to poor digestive processes and a poor immune system.

*Stage 4: the colon (large intestine)*

If you are suffering from an impaired digestion because of an acid/alkaline imbalance in the small intestine, the improperly digested food will pass on into the colon. You may notice that the large intestine is not mentioned in the 'what should' happen section, and for good reason. If all is working well, nutrients are already absorbed by the time they reach the large intestine, and there are no accompanying problems. In reality, however, what usually happens is as follows:

- Think of the colon as a vast chemical and waste re-cycling unit, always looking for usable components which can be put to good purpose – in this case to produce essential B vitamins.
- Problems occur when the large intestine becomes overfilled with undigested food. This allows enemies such as the yeast-like organism Candida albicans to grow and flourish because there aren't enough friendly bacteria to fight them. This imbalance can be made worse by factors in modern life: the good bugs are also depleted by antibiotics (which destroy bad and good indiscriminately) and other pharmaceutical drugs including steroids and the contraceptive Pill, alcohol and high degrees of stress.

## Candida

In moderation, Candida albicans is useful; it's designed to mop up the residue left over when protein and carbohydrates have given over their nutrients in stage 3. Normally there would never be enough food for it to expand beyond its own territory. Given an overfilled colon, however, the Candida romps out of control, becoming what is known medically as 'systemic', and searching out food to fuel its ever expanding form.

In excess candida grows like a spider's web. It stretches out and invades the wall of the large intestine, causing that to become more porous and eventually leading to leaky gut syndrome. This brings with it a crowd of symptoms including head, muscle and joint aches, acute fatigue, nausea, dry skin and skin rashes. As the gut becomes progressively more porous, small particles of protein get into the bloodstream and the body reacts to these allergens by producing histamine. In a vicious circle of reactions, this can lead to the immune system setting up allergic reactions to the allergens (foods), which brings on symptoms such as asthma, skin rashes, migraine and hay fever.

Another possible consequence of yeast overgrowth is gut fermentation. Your large intestine becomes like a vat. The different yeasts produce a range of toxic alcohols all of which must be processed by the liver. In return for its work overload, the liver makes you feel exhausted and lethargic.

So you can see why so many people suffer from a mid-afternoon energy dip, often accompanied by drowsiness and mood swings, after they eat their lunchtime sandwich and cake, just bursting with sugar, yeast and carbohydrates. They are literally feeding a brewery and pouring toxic waste into their bloodstream. The sugars and carbohydrates are fuelling the yeast, and the contents of the sandwich – such as fatty ham or cheese – are suppressing the production and utilisation of bile and enzymes. Not good for a working afternoon, or even having fun.

The solution is simple. Take a good acidophilus supplement to support the intestinal tract (Immunoguard from Biocare is a good choice), and then join the chew, chew cult. It's free and it works.

# ☙ 5

# Desperate Measures: The Seven-Day Weight-Loss Plan

There are times when that extra bulge is just one too many for a special occasion. Usually we advise a slow steady rate of weight loss of one to two pounds (just under 1kg) weekly but in extreme situations – weddings are one of the most common – many readers will be able to accelerate the process safely by following this Seven-Day Weight-Loss plan.

There are a couple of warnings, however:

Firstly, before you do this diet, you should have filled in the questionnaires to identify your Biotype and any Stress Weakness. If you have scored 10 or more in any of the Stress Weakness categories, the probability of this plan working well for you will be reduced. Correct your Stress Weakness before embarking on it (by that stage, you may well have lost the undesired weight anyway).

The second warning is this: however slim they are, some people still see themselves as being fat. While we don't need to tell you the risks linked to obesity (including heart disease and diabetes), neither do we want people to lose more weight than is wise for their body and shape. Very few women are meant to be supermodel thin; equally, men are not designed to weigh the same as a flat race jockey. So before you start, please be careful to establish whether or not you need to lose this amount of weight. You can do this by following the step-by-step instructions below.

## Assessing your weight

### 1. Body Mass Index

An accurate and individualised way to assess your weight is to calculate your Body Mass Index (BMI). This gives you a good picture of whether or not you are under- or overweight, healthy or obese. The only drawback with the BMI is that it does not differentiate between fat and muscle so, in some cases, it is possible that overweight people who are very fit may be more healthy than thin people who are very unfit. To gauge this differential, see the information on Fat Monitors below.

#### How to calculate your Body Mass Index (BMI)
Your BMI is calculated by dividing your weight in pounds by your height in inches squared. If this sounds a nightmare for non-mathematicians, just get on the Net and punch in Body Mass Index and you will find lots of sites that do it for you instantly. You can also get a general guideline from the chart opposite.

Otherwise, find a calculator and follow these instructions.

Write down your weight in pounds, multiply by 703.
Write down your height in inches, then square that figure.
Now divide your weight in pounds by your height in inches squared.

## Body Mass Index Chart

| Height (inches) | Body Weight (pounds) Safe | | | | | | Overweight | | | | | Obese | | | | | |
|---|---|---|---|---|---|---|---|---|---|---|---|---|---|---|---|---|---|
| 58 | 91 | 96 | 100 | 105 | 110 | 115 | 119 | 124 | 129 | 134 | 138 | 143 | 148 | 153 | 158 | 162 | 167 |
| 59 | 94 | 99 | 104 | 109 | 114 | 119 | 124 | 128 | 133 | 138 | 143 | 148 | 153 | 158 | 163 | 168 | 173 |
| 60 | 97 | 102 | 107 | 112 | 118 | 123 | 128 | 133 | 138 | 143 | 148 | 153 | 158 | 163 | 168 | 174 | 179 |
| 61 | 100 | 106 | 111 | 116 | 122 | 127 | 132 | 137 | 143 | 148 | 153 | 158 | 164 | 169 | 174 | 180 | 185 |
| 62 | 104 | 109 | 115 | 120 | 126 | 131 | 136 | 142 | 147 | 153 | 158 | 164 | 169 | 175 | 180 | 186 | 191 |
| 63 | 107 | 113 | 118 | 124 | 130 | 135 | 141 | 146 | 152 | 158 | 163 | 169 | 175 | 180 | 186 | 191 | 197 |
| 64 | 110 | 116 | 122 | 128 | 134 | 140 | 145 | 151 | 157 | 163 | 169 | 174 | 180 | 186 | 192 | 197 | 204 |
| 65 | 114 | 120 | 126 | 132 | 138 | 144 | 150 | 156 | 162 | 168 | 174 | 180 | 186 | 192 | 198 | 204 | 210 |
| 66 | 118 | 124 | 130 | 136 | 142 | 148 | 155 | 161 | 167 | 173 | 179 | 186 | 192 | 198 | 204 | 210 | 216 |
| 67 | 121 | 127 | 134 | 140 | 146 | 153 | 159 | 166 | 172 | 178 | 185 | 191 | 198 | 204 | 211 | 217 | 223 |
| 68 | 125 | 131 | 138 | 144 | 151 | 158 | 164 | 171 | 177 | 184 | 190 | 197 | 203 | 210 | 216 | 223 | 230 |
| 69 | 128 | 135 | 142 | 149 | 155 | 162 | 169 | 176 | 182 | 189 | 196 | 203 | 209 | 216 | 223 | 230 | 236 |
| 70 | 132 | 139 | 146 | 153 | 160 | 167 | 174 | 181 | 188 | 195 | 202 | 209 | 216 | 222 | 229 | 236 | 243 |
| 71 | 136 | 143 | 150 | 157 | 165 | 172 | 179 | 186 | 193 | 200 | 208 | 215 | 222 | 229 | 236 | 243 | 250 |
| 72 | 140 | 147 | 154 | 162 | 169 | 177 | 184 | 191 | 199 | 206 | 213 | 221 | 228 | 235 | 242 | 250 | 258 |
| 73 | 144 | 151 | 159 | 166 | 174 | 182 | 189 | 197 | 204 | 212 | 219 | 227 | 235 | 242 | 250 | 257 | 265 |
| 74 | 148 | 155 | 163 | 171 | 179 | 186 | 194 | 202 | 210 | 218 | 225 | 233 | 241 | 249 | 256 | 264 | 272 |
| 75 | 152 | 160 | 168 | 176 | 184 | 192 | 200 | 208 | 216 | 224 | 232 | 240 | 248 | 256 | 264 | 272 | 279 |
| 76 | 156 | 164 | 172 | 180 | 189 | 197 | 205 | 213 | 221 | 230 | 238 | 246 | 254 | 263 | 271 | 279 | 287 |
| BMI | 19 | 20 | 21 | 22 | 23 | 24 | 25 | 26 | 27 | 28 | 29 | 30 | 31 | 32 | 33 | 34 | 35 |

Weight 145 lbs
multiply by 703
= 101935

Height 67 ins
multiplied by 67
= 4489

Therefore BMI = 101935 divided by 4489 = 22.7

## Scoring

*Under 20:* you are underweight; do not follow the Seven-Day Weight-Loss Plan.

*Between 20 and 24.99:* you're within normal healthy range; you should not be trying to lose weight. If you feel passionate about losing weight (wanting to get into an outfit you wore 10 years ago is not really a good enough reason), check with your doctor before embarking on this diet. Otherwise, your wisest course is to follow your Biotype diet, correct any Stress Weaknesses and take moderate exercise (such as walking, swimming, yoga) to tone your body. After this, you may find you have lost the weight anyway.

*Between 25 and 26.99:* you are overweight and can safely follow the Seven-Day Weight-Loss Plan.

*Between 27 and 29.99:* consult your GP or health professional before embarking on the Seven-Day Weight-Loss Plan.

*Over 30:* this range is medically termed obese; you do need to lose weight, but you should seek qualified medical advice before embarking on any diet.

## 2. Fat monitor

You can also calculate your excess weight by using a Fat Monitor. This is a simple electrical device that can calculate the amount of body fat you are carrying. It works by calculating the rate at which a minute electrical pulse flows through the body, a process called bio-electrical impedance analysis (BIA).

Your cellular structure is mainly salty water, which is a good conductor; body fat is very low in water, and is therefore a poor conductor. The more fat you are carrying, the greater the resistance. Using this principle, the machine can calculate your optimum Body Mass. Most BIA monitors have a memory so that your progress can be stored and compared to previous readings. These devices are not cheap (they range from about £50/$75). The advantage is that they differentiate between fat and muscle, unlike the Body Mass Index, so that you have a more accurate reflection of the fat you need to lose.

---

**Warning**

If you are fitted with a pacemaker, check with your doctor before using a BIA monitor or similar.

---

## The Seven-Day Weight-Loss Plan

The quick weight-loss plan we recommend is a seven-day, no-carbohydrates, no-starch weight-loss programme. This programme works by breaking down the fat reserves stored in the body. To achieve this end, the meat eaters do not eat any carbohydrates, only protein in the form of meat, poultry or fish, plus vegetables and fruit. Vegetarians, however, must eat carefully controlled amounts of protein-rich carbohydrates.

Most people lose 6 pounds (2.5 kg) or more during the seven days. Remember, however, that everyone's response to losing weight is individual. Some Biotypes lose weight more easily than others; Pathfinders and Hunter Gatherers are likely to lose the extra pounds more quickly than Pioneers and Farmer Gardeners. Other factors influence the process, too; if, for instance, you have habitually dieted and then indulged in compensation eating, your body will be used to ignoring dietary changes and you will probably lose only three or four pounds (about 1.5kg).

It is vital that you do not put off eating. Vegetarians should make sure they eat something every three hours: your programme should include breakfast, mid-morning snack, lunch, mid-afternoon snack and early supper (leave at least two hours between your evening meal and going to bed so that your digestion has finished processing the food and will not disturb your sleep), with a small snack before you go to bed if you go to bed late, or feel any munchies coming on. Meat eaters tend not to feel hungry on their weight-loss plan but, if you do, have one of the suggested snacks.

*Never* be tempted to stop eating altogether. You risk long-term damage to your body and your mind in return for a dubious short-term gain. You are also likely to incur un-attractive side-effects, such as bad breath, anxiety, physical jitteriness, insomnia and lack of energy.

### Water water every day – and plenty of juice!

As usual, we emphasise the need to drink plenty of still, pure, room-temperature water and also to drink freshly made organic vegetable and fruit juices daily as part of the programme. The reason is this: you are embarking on what's known as a ketogenic diet – that refers to the breaking down of the body fats and the production of ketones, which are excreted through the urine. The presence of the ketones in the urine can lead to fatigue, sluggishness and headaches. This potential problem can be overcome by juicing – which ensures you have enough nutrients in your system – and also by keeping up your water levels. Your body is made up of between 60 and 70 per cent watery fluid so you must always keep up water intake, especially during this time. Different people need different amounts of water: start with at least one litre of water daily and increase as needed. Some people need three to four litres daily, especially those who work in dehydrated environments such as air-conditioned offices.

### No carbs and no starches

Yes, carbohydrates and starches are the same thing! We just want to remind you that they come under different labels on packets and in recipes.

Below, you will find two seven-day menus, with ideas for meals and snacks that you can mix and match. The first includes meat, poultry and fish; vegetarians who eat poultry and/or fish will be able to follow this. More rigorous vegetarians should go to the second weight-loss plan: this does not contain meat, poultry or fish, but does include cheese (which can, of course, be vegetarian) and eggs, if liked.

## Worst weight offenders

These are listed in order of importance. Those at the top are the worst; those at the bottom are the least bad in terms of weight loss.

- pastry
- croissant
- cookies
- flapjacks, etc.
- cakes
- white bread
- pasta
- potatoes
- black/brown bread
- white rice/ couscous
- brown rice and wholegrains
- muesli
- jacket potatoes

## The plans

Note: remember all products should be organic wherever possible, most importantly meat, poultry and eggs

### Weight-loss plan for meat, poultry and/or fish eaters

**Food categories**

The foods in this plan are divided into three categories:

- Eat as much as you want
- Eat limited amounts
- Don't eat at all while you're following the weight-loss plan

As long as you stick to the lists below, you can eat whatever you like at any meal. The most important thing is to have a hearty breakfast and drink your raw vegetable juice in the morning (see page 174).

## Eat as much as you want of

- Steaks in the form of lean meat, poultry or fish (such as beef, turkey, cod or tuna)
- Roast lamb or lean grilled chops with the fat trimmed off
- Eggs, boiled, poached or fried in 1 tsp olive oil
- Poultry and game, on the bone, minced or pre-sliced
- Fish; white fish and oily fish, fresh, canned or frozen
- Tofu (soya bean curd)
- Raw vegetable juice, see below (the left-over fibre can be cooked with vegetable stock, vegetables and lean meat to make a very filling low-calorie meal)
- Soft fruit: including strawberries, raspberries, currants, kiwi, grapefruit, watermelon (other melon is OK, if you can't get watermelons), peaches, nectarines. Out of season, you can use frozen berries and other fruit but do not use canned fruit because sugar is used as a preservative

## Eat limited amounts of

Each of these foods has an upper daily limit. Try to avoid eating any more than this in any one day.

- Hard cheese, any kind, up to 3oz (75g)
- Full fat organic cream, up to 3 teaspoons (90ml) a day *or* 1 pint (20floz/600ml) of semi-skimmed or skimmed organic milk.
- Low-fat natural yoghurt, preferably live, up to 10floz (300ml)

- Mushrooms, up to 3oz (75g)
- Salads, up to 2 medium-sized bowls of leafy greens, celery, mange tout, cauliflower, broccoli, radishes and cucumber
- Cooked vegetables, up to 2 medium-sized bowls of greens, broccoli, cabbage, spinach, kale, Chinese leaf, courgettes, marrow, cauliflower, mange tout
- Fresh tomato and basil sauce, with no sugar or flour, 2 cups (about 500ml)
- Coffee or tea, up to three cups a day with milk or cream from your daily allowance if wished, but no sugar
- Alcohol, 2 small glasses of dry wine a day (about 8floz in total, or 240ml)

**Don't eat at all (on the weight-loss plan)**

- Any flour or flour-based products
- Any products containing sugar or other forms of sweetener, such as breads, pancakes, cereals, cakes, sweets, spaghetti or pasta
- Jams or preserves of any kind, honey or syrup
- Ice-cream
- Sweetened and/or fruit yoghurts
- Frozen sweetened yoghurts
- Pickles, ketchup or prepared sauces
- Oranges, bananas, pears or grapes
- Peas and root vegetables, including potatoes in any form
- Rice, couscous, whole-grains, muesli or porridge
- Shellfish

**It's OK . . .**

- While using this programme it is perfectly OK to drink both tea and coffee provided that you are drinking organic produce; choose decaffeinated, if possible. You can drink as much herb or ginger tea, bought or homemade, as you like.

- Drink at least one litre of still pure water at room temperature each day.

## Cooking

You have several options for cooking the main dish:

- Meats, poultry and fish: poach, grill or bake
- Vegetables: steam or eat raw (to preserve the nutrients)
- Herbs: Use as many fresh herbs as you can with meals; make food as appealing as possible
- Butter and oil: Allow yourself 1oz (25g) of butter (organic, if possible) daily, either to cook with or as a topping for a dish. Also allow yourself 1 tsp (5ml) of olive (or any other) oil daily, either to cook with, or as a dressing. Alternatively, if you do not use any butter, increase your daily oil allowance to 3 dessertspoonsful (about 45ml)
- Dressings: Use your oil allowance to dress salads, vegetables or to fry in
- Make a flavourful oil by putting a dried chopped chilli and/or a peeled garlic clove and/or a chunk of peeled ginger plus strong Mediterranean herbs (such as basil, rosemary, thyme, oregano) in a bottle and top with good olive (or other) oil. Leave it to stand for a few days, then use this wonderfully flavoured oil on salad or vegetables. Add more oil as the level drops. You can also make a natural yoghurt dressing by mixing the yoghurt with torn fresh herbs and lemon juice. Or make a traditional vinaigrette with 3 parts oil (olive or nut oil) to 1 part vinegar or lemon juice with salt and pepper. Add herbs liberally to

any dressing. You can also use any low calorie ready prepared dressing (organic if possible) provided that it does not contain sugar, sugar substitute or starch in any form. If it contains oil, calculate this as part of your daily allowance. If it is yoghurt–based, do the same.

### First thing

Start each day with a cup of warm water with a squeeze of lemon.

---

### Juice

Many people choose to have their fresh juice first thing in the morning, then follow it with breakfast a little later. To one large glass of raw vegetable juice add two heaped teaspoons of psyllium husk or take 6 capsules of psyllium husk with it. (The psyllium ensures that you have regular bowel movements and also gives you a feeling of being full.)

If you are a non-breakfast person, just have juice first thing but make absolutely certain to eat your breakfast by mid-morning or you may develop the dreaded cookie craving.

Follow the detox diet in the Juice section (see page 189), from days 1 to 5. On days 6 and 7, drink a large glass of the Ultimate Juice every morning.

---

### Breakfast

Some of the following ideas may appeal:

- 1 or 2 hard boiled eggs and 1oz (25g) of hard cheese
- Scrambled eggs made with 2 or 3 eggs, 1 tsp butter and/or 2 tsp cream from your daily allowance, with a 3oz (75g)

serving of mushrooms, cooked in a spot of butter or a teaspoon of oil from your daily allowance and lemon juice, garnished with parsley, coriander or tarragon

- Scrambled eggs made with 2 eggs, garnished with 2oz (50g) chopped smoked salmon and chopped green herbs
- 3oz (75g) block smoked tofu fried in olive oil and herbs with 1 or 2 fried eggs, if liked
- 3–4oz (75–100g) smoked haddock (non-dyed) poached in skimmed milk and water, garnished with parsley
- Kipper (non-dyed), grilled and garnished with parsley
- 1 poached egg, with a 3oz (75g) serving mushrooms, cooked as above
- 4oz (100g) grilled liver, kidney or bacon (or a combination of all three, totalling no more than 4oz/100g
- 1 cup yoghurt (about 250ml) with 6 chopped soaked almonds (soak for 24 hours in water; do not put in fridge) and hazel nuts; topped with ground cinnamon

**Snacks**

Don't eat these unless you are hungry!

- Crudités (any fresh vegetable) with low-calorie dressing (bought or homemade), tzatziki (cucumber and yoghurt dip) or aubergine dip
- Soft fruit
- Beef or salmon jerky

**Lunch and dinner**

Eat as much as you really want. Remember do not add or eat any thickened sauces or root vegetables. Eat slowly and chew your food well. All oil, butter and cream should be taken from your daily allowance.

- Large grilled or roasted lamb or beef steak with all the fat trimmed off, a medium-sized green salad with oil, lemon and herb dressing
- Large serving of chicken, guinea fowl or turkey, with a medium-sized green salad or a small serving of broccoli
- Stir-fried lean chicken or turkey with ginger, sugar snap peas and green beans
- Grilled liver, cauliflower with hard cheese grated over the top (or make a cheese sauce with Gram flour and some of your butter and milk allowance)
- Venison steak fried in oil with mushrooms, garlic and herbs, with sliced yellow, green and red peppers (raw or cooked)
- Grilled or baked plaice, cod or salmon, with steamed green vegetables
- Firm fish (such as coley or cod) stir-fried with sprouted bean shoots, celery, sugar snap peas and watercress
- Grilled halibut or other white fish, courgettes fried in oil allowance with garlic and herbs
- Avocado pear with oil and lemon, poached salmon with fresh tomato sauce, a green leafy salad with oil dressing
- Avocado pear with yoghurt dressing and mixed chopped nuts, tomato salad garnished with chopped herbs, and a green leafy salad with oil dressing
- Smoked organic fish (such as mackerel, trout or salmon) or tinned tuna with tomato and green salad

---

**Top tip**

Try tinned squid or octopus chunks if you're in a hurry – rather like chewy chicken, say our testers.

---

**Desserts**

Most desserts automatically fall on the forbidden list so, if in doubt, don't! However, there are some delicious puds that you can indulge in. Biotypes who are following a food-combining programme should eat fruit puddings one or two hours after a main meal.

Try one of the following:

- Red fruits (redcurrants, strawberries, raspberries – fresh or frozen) with 3 to 4 dessertspoons of sour cream, fromage frais, cottage cheese or yoghurt
- Cubed melon (any variety) in natural low-fat yoghurt with torn fresh mint and/or cinnamon
- Low-fat yoghurt with chopped fresh almonds and torn fresh mint
- Soaked, stewed dried fruit, warm or cold, with sour cream, fromage frais, cottage cheese or yoghurt (substitute rhubarb in season, but not canned)
- Sliced watermelon and kiwi, arranged in overlapping slices on plate, with or without other fresh fruits on the list
- 2 small apples
- 2oz (50g) hard cheese

### Weight-loss plan for vegetarians

Vegetarians have different requirements to meat, poultry and fish eaters when it comes to a fat-burning diet. You must have protein, and the best protein is beans, tofu (or tempeh) and nuts. So there is no denying that it's hard work to make this programme varied. Just remember that the results will justify the tedium. If you eat eggs, you can substitute one hard boiled egg for the protein content of any main meal on alternate days. You will see that cheese is included in some dishes, and strict vegetarians can substitute vegetarian cheese.

If you want to eat exactly the same meals each day from Days 1 to 4, and 6 and 7, do so. You will, however, see that Day 5 is different, for the reasons explained below, and you must stick to that. The most important thing is to have a hearty breakfast and to drink your raw vegetable juice in the morning (see page 174).

**Food categories**

The foods in this plan are divided into three categories:

- Eat as much as you want
- Eat limited amounts
- Don't eat at all while you're following the weight-loss plan

**Eat as much as you want of**

- Tofu (soya bean curd)
- Quorn (a mushroom mycoprotein)
- Raw vegetable juice, see below (the left over fibre can be cooked with vegetable stock, vegetables and vegetable protein to make a very filling low-calorie meal)
- Soft fruit, including strawberries, raspberries, currants, kiwi, grapefruit, watermelon (other melons are OK if you can't get watermelons), peaches and nectarines. Out of season, you can use frozen berries and other fruit, but do not use canned fruit because sugar is used as a preservative

**Eat limited amounts of**

Each of these foods has an upper daily limit. Try to avoid eating any more than this in any one day.

- Fresh mixed nuts – almond, hazel, walnut, pecan, pistachio (do not eat dry roasted, salted or glazed), up to 6oz (150g)
- Hard cheese, any kind, up to 3oz (75g)
- Full fat organic cream – up to 3 teaspoons a day, or 1 pint (20floz/600ml) of semi-skimmed/skimmed organic milk
- Low fat natural yoghurt, preferably live, up to 10floz (300ml)
- Mushrooms, up to 3oz (75g)
- One red, yellow or green pepper daily, or that amount in different colours
- Salads: up to 2 medium-sized bowls of leafy greens, celery, mange tout, cauliflower, broccoli, radishes and cucumber
- Cooked vegetables, up to 2 medium-sized bowls of greens, broccoli, cabbage, spinach, kale, Chinese leaf, courgettes, marrow, cauliflower and mange tout
- Fresh tomato and basil sauce, with no sugar or flour, up to 2 cups (about 500ml)
- Coffee or tea, up to 3 cups a day, with milk or cream from your daily allowance if wished, but no sugar
- Alcohol, 2 small glasses of dry wine a day (about 8floz in total, or 240ml)

**Don't eat at all (on the weight-loss plan)**

- Any flour or flour-based products
- Any products containing sugar or other forms of sweetener, such as breads, pancakes, cereals, cakes, sweets, spaghetti or pasta
- Jams or preserves of any kind, honey or syrup
- Ice-cream
- Sweetened and/or fruit yoghurts
- Frozen sweetened yoghurts
- Pickles, ketchup or prepared sauces

- Oranges, bananas, pears or grapes
- Peas and root vegetables, including potatoes in any form
- Rice, couscous, whole-grains, muesli or porridge

## It's OK . . .

- While using this programme it is perfectly OK to drink both tea and coffee provided that you are drinking organic products; choose decaffeinated, if possible. You can drink as much herb or ginger tea, bought or homemade, as you like
- Drink at least one litre of still pure water at room temperature each day

## Cooking

You have several options for cooking the main dish:

- Vegetables: steam or eat raw (to preserve the nutrients)
- Tofu: flash fry with 1 tsp garlic or other flavoured oil, steam or bake with herbs (see Recipes, page 228)
- Quorn: as directed on packet
- Herbs: use as many fresh herbs as you can with meals; make food as appealing and colourful as possible
- Butter: this is not allowed at all during this week
- Oil: allow yourself three dessertspoonfuls (about 45ml) of olive (or any other) oil daily
- Dressings: use your oil allowance to dress salads, vegetables or to fry in
- Make a flavourful oil by putting a dried chopped chilli and/or a peeled garlic clove and/or a chunk of peeled ginger plus strong Mediterranean herbs (such as basil, rosemary, thyme, oregano) in a bottle and top with good olive (or other) oil. Leave it to stand for a few days, then use

this wonderfully flavoured oil on salad or vegetables. Add more oil as the level drops. You can also make a natural yoghurt dressing by mixing the yoghurt with torn fresh herbs and lemon juice. Or make a traditional vinaigrette with 3 parts oil (olive or nut oil) to 1 part vinegar or lemon juice with salt and pepper. Add herbs liberally to any dressing. You can also use any low calorie ready prepared dressing (organic if possible) provided that it does not contain sugar, sugar substitute or starch in any form. If it contains oil, calculate this as part of your daily allowance. If it is yoghurt-based, do the same.

- Nuts: if possible, never consume salted or dry roasted nuts; buy fresh, shell-on nuts. Soaking them in water for 24 hours, or steaming them, releases the protein and makes it more bio-available.

**First thing**
Start each day with a cup of warm water with a squeeze of lemon.

---

**Juice**

Many people choose to have their fresh juice first thing in the morning, then follow it with breakfast a little later. To one large glass of raw vegetable juice, add two heaped teaspoons of psyllium husk or take 6 capsules of psyllium husk with it. (The psyllium ensures that you have regular bowel movements and also gives you a feeling of being full.)

If you are a non-breakfast person, just have juice but make absolutely certain to eat your breakfast by mid-morning or you may develop the dreaded cookie craving.

---

Follow the detox diet in the Juice section (see page 189), from days 1 to 5. On days 6 and 7, drink a large glass of the Ultimate Juice every morning.

### Days 1 to 4

**Breakfast**

Choose from one of the following ideas:

- 4floz (120ml) of low-fat yoghurt with 2oz (50g) of fresh/frozen soft fruits or berries such as strawberries, raspberries, loganberries, redcurrants, blackcurrant and gooseberries, with 1 teaspoon molasses, if wished
- 3oz (75g) of fresh fruit, such as satsuma, pear, apple, nectarine, pink grapefruit, orange, plum, persimmon covered with 5floz (150ml) low-fat yoghurt and 1 teaspoon of molasses, if wished
- 6oz (150g) of melon (any type) cubes with low-fat live natural yoghurt
- 1 carton of soya yoghurt with 2oz (50g) chopped fresh nuts and a teaspoon of molasses

**Snacks**

Ideas for mid-morning and mid-afternoon snacks:

- 2 small apples
- 2oz (50g) of freshly shelled, mixed nuts.
- 1 8floz (250ml) fruit smoothie, using any fruits apart from bananas and grapes; blend with some ice cubes to make it thick and frosty cold
- 2oz (50g) walnuts and pecans
- 2 pieces of fruit from the following list: pear, persimmon,

plum, nectarine, fig, date, orange, pink grapefruit and satsuma (but do not eat more than one piece of citrus fruit)

### Lunch

- 2 tofu burgers with large mixed green salad
- 8oz (200g) Quorn fillets, steamed vegetables, such as carrots, courgettes, broccoli, cauliflower, Savoy cabbage and asparagus, with 2oz (50g) grated hard cheese
- Large mixed salad with 2oz (50g) mixed beans, either tinned or soaked and cooked, such as pinto, butter beans, haricot beans, flageolet, soya beans, chickpeas and lima beans
- 8oz (200g) sprouted beans and bean shoots, steamed or stir-fried in 1 tsp olive oil, with 1oz (25g) parmesan cheese or any other hard cheese (vegetarian if wished)
- 1 large egg (alternate days only), hard-boiled, with low-calorie dressing, if wished, with medium-sized bowl of mixed salad

### Dinner

- 2oz (50g) of beans such as pinto, butter beans, haricot beans, flageolet, soya beans, chickpeas, lima beans either tinned or soaked and cooked, with low-calorie dressing
- 8oz (200g) of mixed green salad
- 2oz (50g) of mixed beans
- 8oz (200g) salad of mixed red peppers, green peppers, yellow peppers, beetroot, bean shoots, fennel and fresh mint, with low-calorie dressing
- 8oz (200g) of steamed vegetables such as carrots, courgettes, broccoli, cauliflower, Savoy cabbage and asparagus topped with 1oz (25g) of chopped, soaked almonds and/or

walnuts and 1oz (25g) grated fresh parmesan or other hard cheese

- 4oz (100g) steamed white fish *or* a 6oz (150g) block of tofu or Quorn fillet, 6oz (150g) steamed vegetables, such as courgettes, broccoli, cauliflower, Savoy cabbage, asparagus, fennel, celery, spinach, onions and marrow
- Large platter of mixed crudités (any type of vegetable), with 2 tsp guacamole, 2 tsp hummus and 2 tsp tzatziki
- Large platter of roasted vegetables, such as red and yellow peppers, courgettes, mushrooms, asparagus, leeks and aubergines, with 1oz (25g) fresh parmesan or other hard cheese (slice with potato peeler in long slivers)

**Desserts**
- 2oz (50g) soft fruits, such as strawberries, raspberries, logan-berries, blackberries and mulberries, with sour cream, fromage frais, yoghurt or cottage cheese
- 2oz (50g/dry weight) stewed mixed dried fruits, such as figs, dates, prunes, apricots, pears, peaches and coconut, with sour cream, fromage frais, yoghurt or cottage cheese

## Day 5: Little and often

On the fifth day, vegetarians need to eat small amounts of food at two-hourly intervals because this is the day when most people get a mad urge to eat non-stop. That's because the body is actually changing the way it handles food and your brain is reacting by trying to go back to what it knows. By topping up through the little-and-often grazing programme below, you can keep your body and brain happy. At no point should you feel hungry.

*Waking*
- A glass of still mineral water with a squeeze of fresh lemon juice

*Breakfast*
- The fifth juice in the detox programme
- 1 small (5floz/150ml) soya yoghurt with 1 tsp black-strap molasses

*10am*
- 1oz (25g) of your favourite nuts (from the nuts list on page 179)

*Midday*
- 2 pieces of your favourite fruit (from the fruit list on page 178)

*2pm*
- medium-sized green salad with oil dressing and 1oz (25g) grated cheese

*4pm*
- 1 sweet eating apple and 1oz (25g) walnuts or pecans

*6pm*
- 1 pink grapefruit as a smoothie or eaten whole

*8pm*
- 6oz (150g) steamed vegetables with a flavoured olive oil dressing

*10pm and beyond*
- If you're going to keep going at this point, eat 1oz (25g) dried fruit, with a medium-sized glass of still mineral water until you go to bed

### Days 6 and 7

Follow the programme for days 1 to 4.

## 🐚 6

# Get Juicing

Once you get gripped by juicing, you will wonder how you ever got by without this natural fountain of youth. Fresh vegetable and fruit juices are supercharged nourishment in highly concentrated liquid form. People who formerly looked pallid, podgy and tired start knocking back a raw energy cocktail daily and Abracadabra! they're transformed into vital energetic human beings with bright healthy skin and eyes. Juicing is quite simply the cheapest and most effective long-term strategy for maintaining your health at every age and stage.

As well as being a wonderful addition to your life in general, juices are an indispensable part of the Seven-Day Weight-Loss Plan (see Chapter 5). Juiced raw vegetables are high in natural vitamins, minerals and plant enzymes. There is no food or food product that can provide the same amount of vital nutrients at such a low cost. And no single vitamin or mineral supplement has such a synergistic balance of the essential components needed to keep you healthy. Incidentally, Norman Walker, the man who pioneered juicing in America, died at the ripe old age of 113.

Juicing has a long and honoured history in the annals of naturopathic and complementary health practices. It was the basis of many early so-called 'miracle' cures, probably because the concentration of antioxidants and other essential vitamins and minerals flooding through the system in high doses can have a radical effect on some illness. Juices help to detox your body and, simultaneously, to stimulate the immune system and other functions.

Drunk first thing in the morning, fresh juices kickstart your metabolism into working joyously. Try the Adam & Eve Ultimate Juice Formula, or our other recipes, or experiment with your own combinations.

Always drink your fresh juice immediately; the fresher the juice, the more vitality there is in the mixture. The taste of freshly juiced vegetables is often very different to that of raw vegetables. Beetroot, for instance, is sweet and celery has a milder tang. Although bottles of ready-made juice may have some nutrients (as well as some chemical additives – in non-organic juices – that you would rather not have), they have been pasteurised (boiled to kill bacteria and disease organisms) to ensure shelf life, so there is absolutely no comparison to the nutrients in fresh juices.

If you are trying to give up nicotine, coffee or alcohol you'll find that juicing is a great help. By giving your body a morning 'hit', you can often avoid the craving for your banned substance.

The only drawback is that they take a little bit of time to make – perhaps 10 minutes in all – by the time you have prepared the vegetables and forced them through the feed tube. You can, of course, go and buy them freshly made at many organic stores, but that's expensive on a daily basis – and besides, you have to get dressed and go out. So bite the juice bullet: invest in a juicer and get up and glow.

> 'Raw juice is the most perfect fuel for your body. Fresh juices are bursting with life power, a natural raw energy that is miraculous in its beneficial effect on the human body.'
>
> Leslie Kenton, author and devoted juicer for 35 years

## The Five-Day Juice Detox

The Adam & Eve juice regime is designed to detoxify at progressively deeper levels over five days. Starting with the basic melon and celery formula on Day 1, which is full of antioxidant vitamins (principally vitamins A, C and E) and other nutrients, then working up to the Day 5 vegetable juice, which gives you a deep tissue cleanse. Finally, the Ultimate Juice formula contains a broad spectrum of vegetables and is a general detoxifier that also stimulates the system.

Some readers may wonder why we have not included wheatgrass. This is partly because many people find it so disgusting that they actually gag on it, due to the effect of the chlorophyll on the liver. Virtually all of the nutrients in wheatgrass can be found in the Ultimate Juice formula. However, if you like wheat grass, by all means include it.

There are several ways in which you can incorporate juices into your Biotype diet.

- Have a juice before breakfast everyday
- Add juice to your Seven-Day Weight-Loss Plan
- Follow a juice cleanse by replacing one meal a day with a juice; this should be the evening meal if possible
- Do a one-day fast, replacing meals with juices; this is best done when you have a day of rest, so use it as an opportunity to spoil yourself

---

**Top tips**

- Don't gulp these nourishing juices, sip them. Think of them as soup rather than squash or water.
- Use your juicer to make single fresh fruit juices, such as apple or pear, melon or berry, which you can top up with fizzy spring water and flavour with mint instead of buying soft drinks.

---

### How to make fresh juices

- Wash the raw vegetables under cold running water
- Scrub any root vegetables
- Peel thick-skinned fruit, such as pineapple, melon, citrus fruit and kiwi
- Stone cherries, peaches, etc.
- Avoid using fibrous fruit, such as bananas, rhubarb and apricots because they don't give very much juice and clog up the juicer
- Chop fruit and vegetables in small enough sections to fit through your feeder tube without getting stuck (this is usually the most irritating part)
- Roll up leaf vegetables tightly
- Put parsley, celery, and any other leafy-ended vegetables in stem end first
- Place in the juicer

---

'Juice makes you feel good. It is a gone-in-a-minute glass of vital, power-packed liquid that will make you feel 20 years younger.'

Nigel Slater, The *Observer* Magazine

---

### Buying a juicer

You will use your juicer as often as you use your coffee maker and it has to stand up to tough treatment, so buy the best you can afford. The price range is wide – from around £30 to over £300. Having said that, we both have Kenwood juicers that cost under £50 and while they are a bit fiddly, they do the job just fine.

There are three types of juicers:

- Centrifugal juicers use a circular filter basket with fine grating teeth to shred the fruit and vegetables. When they're spun rapidly, centrifugal force separates the juice from the skin, pulp and pips. These juicers are invariably cheaper to buy but give you less juice
- Masticating juicers 'chew' the fruit and vegetables; they are more powerful, usually produce more juice, and they are also much more expensive
- Trituration juicers, the latest generation, crush the vegetables and fruit (including the cell walls); they are quieter, most expensive and the most effective because they extract the maximum nutrients

For more information, see the Directory, page 283

---

### Pink goddess

Not so much a juice as a watermelon!

For the quickest most delicious pink drink with maximum antioxidant vitamins, blend a quarter of a watermelon, seeds and all, with a handful of fresh mint leaves. Add a couple of ice cubes if you wish.

---

### Adam & Eve juices

We have not given precise quantities for the juices. This is because individual juicers vary so much in the amount they give. You will be able to gauge the quantity your juicer gives when you have used it for a week or so. As a rough guide, four large apples, four large carrots and a one inch chunk of ginger give about a third of a pint (8floz/240ml) of juice in our Kenwood juicers.

**Day 1**
Melon (watermelon if possible, otherwise any sort) and celery
  Use a ratio of 3:1, melon to celery, by weight.

- Melon contains beta-carotene, folic acid, vitamin B5, vitamin C, traces of vitamins B1, B2, B3, B6; calcium, magnesium, phosphorus, potassium, sodium; traces of copper, iron and zinc
- Celery contains folic acid, vitamins C, B1, B2, B3, B5, B6, biotin, vitamin E; calcium, chlorine, manganese, phosphorus, potassium, sodium and sulphur

**Day 2**
Celery and apple
  Use a ratio of 1:1, celery to apple, by weight

- Celery contains folic acid, vitamins C, B1, B2, B3, B5, B6, biotin, vitamin E; calcium, chlorine, manganese, phosphorus, potassium, sodium and sulphur
- Apples contain beta-carotene, folic acid, vitamins C, B1, B2, B3, B6, biotin, vitamin E; calcium, chlorine, magnesium, phosphorus, potassium, sulphur; traces of zinc and copper

**Day 3**

Apple and carrot with ginger to taste
Use a ratio of 1:1, apple to carrot, by weight

- Apples contain beta-carotene, folic acid, vitamins C, B1, B2, B3, B6, biotin, vitamin E; calcium, chlorine, magnesium, phosphorus, potassium, sulphur; traces of zinc and copper
- Carrots contains beta-carotene, folic acid, vitamins C, B1, B2, B3, B5, B6, biotin, vitamin E; calcium, chlorine, magnesium, phosphorus, potassium, sodium, sulphur; traces of copper, iron and zinc

---

'When I had my first full glass of fresh juice my entire body came to life instantly. It was as if electricity shot through my veins and instantly I felt better.'

Willard Van De Bogart, quoted in *Alternative Medicine*

---

**Day 4**

Carrot, celery and winter cabbage (or parsley, broccoli, spinach or chard)
Use a ratio of 2 parts carrots and celery stalks, to 1 part cabbage or parsley by weight

- Carrots contains beta-carotene, folic acid, vitamins C, B1, B2, B3, B5, B6, biotin, vitamin E; calcium, chlorine, magnesium, phosphorus, potassium, sodium, sulphur; traces of copper, iron and zinc
- Celery contains folic acid, vitamins C, B1, B2, B3, B5, B6, biotin, vitamin E; calcium, chlorine, manganese, phosphorus, potassium, sodium and sulphur

- Winter cabbage contains folic acid, vitamin C, low levels of B1, B2, B3, B5, B6, biotin and vitamin E; calcium, chlorine, magnesium, phosphorus, potassium, sodium; traces of copper, iron and zinc

---

'I frequently recommend drinking fresh organic juice to my patients and I have heard some amazing stories from them about how it has helped with all sorts of illnesses, including colds, allergies, irritable bowel syndrome, headaches, arthritis and period pain.'

Dr Charles Innes, medical homeopath

---

### Day 5
Carrot, celery, watercress, winter cabbage (or parsley, broccoli, spinach or chard), apple and ginger

Use equal parts of each with ginger to taste (try a one-inch/2.5cm peeled chunk)

- Carrots contains beta-carotene, folic acid, vitamins C, B1, B2, B3, B5, B6, biotin, vitamin E; calcium, chlorine, magnesium, phosphorus, potassium, sodium, sulphur; traces of copper, iron and zinc
- Celery contains folic acid, vitamins C, B1, B2, B3, B5, B6, biotin, vitamin E, calcium, chlorine, manganese, phosphorus, potassium, sodium and sulphur
- Watercress contains beta-carotene, vitamins C and E, low concentrations of B1, B2, B3, B5, B6, biotin; calcium, chlorine, iron, magnesium, phosphorus, potassium, sodium, sulphur; traces of copper and zinc
- Winter cabbage contains folic acid, vitamin C, low levels

of B1, B2, B3, B5, B6; biotin and vitamin E, calcium, chlorine, magnesium, phosphorus, potassium, sodium; traces of
copper, iron and zinc

- Apples contain beta–carotene, folic acid, vitamins C, B1, B2,
B3, B6, biotin, vitamin E; calcium, chlorine, magnesium,
phosphorus, potassium, sulphur; traces of zinc and copper

### The ultimate juice formula

Remember that you can drink this juice any time of the day
– not just in the mornings.

> 2 carrots (make sure you cut off the top end)
> 2 handfuls of sprouted bean shoots
> 4 to 6 stalks celery
> 1/2 small beetroot (make sure you cut off the top end)
> Small handful of parsley or watercress
> Handful of spinach or other dark green vegetable in
>     season, on rotating basis, such as spinach, chard,
>     Savoy cabbage, beet tops, broccoli, etc.
> 1 apple, cooking apple or pear
> Ginger (try a one-inch/2.5cm peeled chunk)

- Watercress contains beta–carotene, vitamins C and E, low
concentrations of vitamins B1, B2, B3, B5, B6, biotin;
calcium, chlorine, iron, magnesium, phosphorus, potassium,
sodium, sulphur; traces of copper and zinc
- Beetroot contains folic acid, vitamin C, low concentrations
of vitamins B1, B2, B3, B5; calcium, magnesium, phosphorus, potassium, sodium; traces of copper, iron and zinc
- Parsley contains beta–carotene, vitamin B3, low concentrations of vitamins B1 and B2; calcium, iron, phosphorus,
potassium and sodium
- Pear contains beta–carotene, folic acid, vitamin C, low

concentrations of vitamins B1, B2, B3, B5, B6; calcium, magnesium, phosphorus, potassium; traces of copper, iron, manganese and zinc

---

## Top tips

- For colds and flu, add a peeled one-inch (2.5cm) chunk of ginger, a large clove of garlic and three black peppercorns to any of the juices; the effect on the symptoms can be dramatic.
- Use the leftover fibre from these juices as the basis of a thick vegetable stock. Put it in a soup pan with some water to cover. Simmer for about an hour, making sure there is enough liquid – add more water if not. Then strain and use as stock for soups or stews.

# ৰ 7

# Relaxation

One of the most common times to reach for comfort food is when you are hot and bothered – under some form of stress in other words. As we explained in Chapter 3, learning how to relax is an indispensable part of coping with your Stress Weaknesses. The way to do it is completely free and very effective. You use your mind and your body to help each other.

Your mind is very powerful and can lift you instantly out of many difficult or painful situations and into a state where you feel calm and secure. Equally, using your body in the right way can help still your mind. Start with the simplest exercise of all – breathing. As you read this, sit up straight (or stand), uncross your arms and legs, let your weight travel towards the floor, and take 6 deep, slow breaths. Breathe in through your nose and out through your mouth. As you inhale, let your stomach swell up with the air like a balloon. Don't let your shoulders rise – imagine your shoulder blades sinking down. As you exhale, feel your tummy shrinking towards your spine.

That's the beginning.

Now think of bringing your mind down from whatever heights it's whizzing around and into your body so that you are functioning as an integrated whole, rather than literally being all over the place. The aim is to bring your anxiety down and with it your blood pressure.

Think down to your navel and start humming from it. Nothing energetic, just a long soft low note that comes from your chest and stomach. You can do this anywhere: it's wonderful in the car, for instance, when road rage is roaring around you.

At home, try meditating. Hunter Gatherers, Farmers and Dancers find it relatively simple to sit down and quieten themselves, and they will find the following method quite easy to do with a bit of practice. Pioneers and Pathfinders, the most physically active of the types, may find they are better suited to chanting, listening to or 'conducting' music (see below), or walking gently through the park. Choose whatever appeals to you.

---

### The Mozart effect

Music soothes. There are bags of evidence showing that music can help heal conditions from migraine to heart disease, insomnia to Parkinson's. Although any music that you like works, listening to Mozart is particularly effective. According to research, Mozart's compositions can calm us, sharpen our IQs and improve concentration, among a crowd of other benefits.

- Play your favourite music anywhere that you become stressed
- Take sing-along tapes/CDs on journeys
- Dispel mental and physical tension by conducting classical (or other) music. If you can conduct properly, do so; but if you can't, just make as if. Put your self wholeheartedly into connecting with all the different strands of the music and the players.

---

- Play the plates! If you happen to have a couple of paper plates handy, you can accompany any music by playing them like cymbals – bases together, shoosh them up and down, side to side, in big and small circles. (Do not take this seriously . . .)
- Lie down on the floor when you're tired, knees bent a hip-width apart, feet flat and pointing forward, head propped on a paperback, hands loosely resting on your navel. Close your eyes and listen to your favourite piece of Mozart, or other music; let your brain follow the music, but don't put effort into this or you will defeat the object. If you start fretting, just gently bring yourself back to the notes. Try to let the music wash into you.
- The brain alters its timing according to the rhythm it hears, so use Gregorian chants, for instance, to calm your brain into sleep, or speedy compositions like the Sabre Dance when you need to speed up a bit.

## Meditation

When you get used to meditating you can do it anywhere, any time, but that may take a bit of practice. Start with a couple of minutes at a time, once or twice a day – early morning and last thing at night are helpful – then gradually increase the time. Remember that there is no correct or incorrect way to do it, whatever suits you is fine.

Here are some simple guidelines:

- Don't meditate when you're feeling hungry, have a full tummy or if you are longing to go to the loo.
- When you first start meditating, find a quiet spot where you won't be interrupted; shut the door and make sure the phone won't ring.

- If this feels appropriate, light a candle and/or say a prayer and/or be grateful to whatever force gave you life.

- Sit comfortably, your feet (bare, if possible) planted firmly on the floor, hands in your lap; uncross your arms and legs, straighten your spine and think of your body softening from crown to toe.

- Breathe deeply, gently, rhythmically; in through your nose and out through your mouth. Make the out breath as long as the in breath. Allow your breathing to fall into a natural rhythm.

- You can meditate simply by focusing on your breathing. Your brain will absorb the rhythm and quieten down. Feel the air as it enters your nostrils, and moves down to fill your lungs completely. Be careful not to let your shoulders rise at this point.

- Breathe in to a count of 4, then let your breath hover for a beat or two – just as a wave hovers on the shore before ebbing away – then exhale to a count of 4. Build up the exhalation until it takes 8 beats.

- Try to breathe from the abdomen rather than the chest and feel your stomach swell as you inhale – rather like a balloon – then flatten again as you exhale.

- If you are tense, imagine every part of your body relaxing; starting with your scalp and hairline, soften every feature of your face then move down slowly through your body, feeling the tension ebb away from neck, shoulders, shoulderblades and spine, stomach, arms, fingers, feet and finally toes.

- If your mind is dogged with invading thoughts, or a loop tape of some tense situation continuously plays in your mind, focus on one neutral or calmly pleasant thing – the colour blue, for example, a cloudless sky, the sea, a clear blue gem, mountain tops or a sunset. Or choose a soothing word and repeat it slowly, over and over again in your mind. If a distracting thought breaks in, simply acknowledge it and let it go. See the thought as a cloud and watch it float away in your mind's eye.

## Creative visualisation

Visualisation uses the same general principles as meditation. With visualisation, however, you are going to focus on creating healing pictures in your mind as well as using other senses. These mind pictures can come in many forms. Here are some ideas. You can also try and identify your own favourites.

- When you feel flustered, think of a place where you have felt happy, secure and calm: a garden in the summer, a gentle beach where you can see the sea disappearing into the horizon, a meadow full of wild flowers.
- Now feel the warmth of the sun on your face, the breeze in your hair, smell the sea or the scent of the flowers, hear the waves or grasses as the wind rustles them.
- Let your mind and body sink into the 'film' in your mind and let go of the problems of the day.
- If a problem bedevils you as you try to sleep, visualise it shut away for the night. This technique is used by Olympic sportsmen. Put the problem in a file, put the file in a drawer, lock the drawer and put the key away. You can do this at any time you want to switch off but the deal is that you must sort out the problem at the next practical opportunity.
- If your left (organising) brain is on overdrive and you can't stop your mind whirring, try crossing over to your right (creative) brain. Do this by focusing your mind in your left

brain; now imagine you are turning away from your left brain and going along a path to your right brain. Go through a door – visualise the details of the door, the colour, shape and texture – turn the handle, open the door then shut it firmly behind you. Explore the place where you find yourself: a walled garden, perhaps, or a peaceful room. Make yourself comfortable – do nothing at all, just exist.

- If you're frightened or uncomfortable, try winding a soft lavender-coloured cocoon around you, from top to bottom, until you are entirely safe. Or, like actress Amanda Burton (a Dancer Biotype), imagine your guardian angels folding their wings around you.

---

### Giving up gracefully

OK, we know giving up is hard to do; we've done it. Cutting down is, too. We also know that giving up substances that don't suit you – alcohol, cigarettes, sugar, or whatever – makes you feel infinitely better. The key to giving up anything is to understand the fighting going on in your mind. While your conscious mind is able to appreciate the reasons for giving up and may be quite prepared to do it, your powerful preconscious mind does not feel the same way. Of course, you can and will give up, it reassures you. Just not today. Giving up gracefully is winning the battle with your preconscious mind.

There is of course a difference between habit and addiction. If you believe you are addicted to a substance of any kind, start by ringing the relevant self-help organisation (see Directory, page 278). Also ask your health practitioner for help.

---

Giving up the habit:

- Set a date; if you suffer from PMS, aim for mid-cycle.
- Write down the reasons for giving up. Be honest about your feelings about the issue.
- Make a list of the benefits and estimate how much giving up (or cutting down) cigs, booze, chocolates will save you. Plan what to do with the money.
- Keep a temptation diary so that you know when you are most vulnerable. Think of distractions to get you through or put yourself in situations where you can't indulge. For example, there's almost nothing else you can do in a sauna or the steam room at the gym, when you're having a massage, on the treadmill, or making love.
- Take up a new hobby that you really want to do.
- Spend time with supportive friends. If you are giving up alcohol or cigarettes and someone constantly tries to tempt you, they are not being supportive.
- It's different if you are cutting down on something like sugar; if you have an overwhelming fancy for something sweet – cake or ice-cream, say – eat a piece of fruit and wait half an hour. If the urge is still irresistible, it's almost always better to have a little and concentrate on really enjoying it. Two mouthfuls of pudding is not going to harm you but try and avoid eating half the cheesecake.
- Remember that whatever you are giving up or cutting down on, you are only doing it for one day at a time. If you want to drink, smoke or binge on ice-cream tomorrow you can. If you reach the end of today and you've stuck to your guns, you're a winner.

## Aromatherapy

We've never met anyone who didn't enjoy relaxing into a bath scented with sweet-smelling essential oils. There is also considerable evidence that aromatherapy has discernible effects that may make it more than simply a very pleasurable experience.

London-based aromatherapist Leigh Richmond has devised these blends especially for the five different Biotypes. We like to use organic oils, such as those by Neal's Yard (see page 282).

For a bath oil, add the recommended number of drops as the taps are running. Alternatively, use the same amount in a room burner or add to distilled water in a spray and mist around a room. For a full body massage, blend into 20 ml of base oil (almond, peach kernel or grapeseed).

### Pathfinders

*Rosemary (4 drops)*

> empowering: strengthens sense of purpose, both individual and collective; inspires boldness and brings clarity

*Pine (8 drops)*

> eases muscular aches and pains; sharpens memory and power of recall

*Lemon (2 drops)*

> detoxifies and purifies the blood; stimulates the brain and helps focus

*Black pepper (2 drops )*

> warms the constitution and eliminates doubts and worries

**Hunter gatherers**

*Sandalwood (4 drops)*

> relates to the throat chakra and so enhances self-expression and effective communication; deeply grounding and comforting; brings balance and a sense of being rooted, which is helpful in a nomadic lifestyle

*Cinnamon (2 drops)*

> invigorating; creates the impetus for adventure and sparks the desire to live life fully

*Basil (4 drops)*

> gives courage in the face of adversity; stimulates fearlessness and boundless optimism, as well as a desire to forge ahead and break new ground

**Pioneers**

*Cedarwood (4 drops)*

> stabilising, empowering; reinforces and strengthens resolve

*Palmarosa (4 drops)*

> encourages adaptability and flexibility so helping to overcome problems such as being stuck in rut or weighed down by responsibility

*Cardamom (2 drops)*

> strengthens resolve and gives a hearty appetite

**Farmer gardeners**

*Ginger (4 drops)*

> warming, caring, abundant; strengthens the constitution

*Juniper (4 drops)*
> helps caregivers to cope with the pressures of other people's problems, but doesn't detract from their strong sense of empathy

*Angelica (2 drops)*
> strengthens the heart and helps to 'heal the healer'

**Dancers**

*Vetivert (4 drops)*
> known as the 'oil of tranquillity'; grounding and soothing, helping to conquer obstacles and calm nervous system

*Chamomile (4 drops) (not in pregnancy)*
> calms hypersensitivity; quells tendency to excess and/or compulsive behaviour

*Immortel (2 drops)*
> a deeply spiritual oil that helps to still mental gymnastics and allows the user to see the bigger picture

## Brain space

You are not a machine. You need rest and relaxation. Plan holidays and put them in the diary. If you are tired, don't push yourself beyond your capabilities; take time off. It may be difficult to take a week, or even a whole day off but most people can manage a half day. So award yourself whatever time off you can – just for you. Do what you want to do. And if that's staying in bed with a novel, that's just fine. Or do something that will enhance your life, such as visiting a picture gallery, seeing a film or having a massage. It need not cost anything at all: sometimes lying on the grass on a sunny day watching the birds wheeling in the sky is the biggest treat possible.

---

### Small change, big difference

Note stress points in your day and consider how you can reduce the pressure. Simple things such as finding a place for your keys, filling up the petrol tank before it hits zero, sorting your clothes cupboard or turning the phone off for an hour when you're trying to concentrate can make a big difference.

---

## Good nights

Many doctors are now convinced that lack of sleep is one of our greatest ills. As well as affecting us physically, it influences our brains and our state of mind. The most helpful asset for good sleep is not pills but a peaceful mind, so if you have a sleeping problem, consider your life in general. Dealing with stress can transform the way you sleep.

### Tips for good sleep

- Try and get to bed before 10pm at least twice a week.
- Do not watch disturbing or over-exciting TV programmes before bed
- Don't have a heavy meal late in the evening; your digestion will keep you awake or disturb you in the night; eat at least two hours before going to bed and don't have heavy rich food; always walk for a short while after the evening meal, in or out of the house

- If you suffer from insomnia, do not drink any caffeinated drinks after midday; preferably cut them out altogether
- Do not eat or drink anything sweet or sugary in the evening; sugar rushes are a prime cause of insomnia
- If you like to have a hot bath at night, make certain that you allow at least half an hour before bed for your body to resume its natural temperature
- Always keep a glass of still water by your bed; one of the most common problems is dehydration which not only wakes you in a state of anxiety but may give you bad dreams
- Keep your bedroom well-ventilated so that you have plenty of oxygen for the night, especially if there is more than one person in the bedroom; if you cannot open your windows, make sure that the door/s are wide
- Make sure your bed and bedclothes are comfortable and pleasing to you; change the mattress every 10 years at least, and turn it regularly; make sure your pillows are comfortable; if you have coloured sheets and are disturbed by them, invest in a new set of white ones
- If you tend to suffer from a stiff neck, shoulders or back when you wake up, never sleep on more than one squishy pillow
- Make your bedroom as peaceful as possible in terms of decoration; also make sure that your curtains and blinds screen out all the light
- If there is any extraneous noise – from snoring partners to noisy neighbours – reduce it as much as possible and use ear plugs
- Do not have electronic gadgets (including TV, computers, music systems or some alarm clocks) in your bedroom, which may emit radiation that agitates the brain

- If you are sleeping with a partner, have two duvets or blankets so that you can keep to the temperature that suits you; preferably also have separate mattresses so that neither of you is disturbed by the other
- Practise a simple breathing routine in bed; simply breathe as in the meditation exercise earlier, visualising waves going up the shore, if you wish
- Play gentle music; there are compositions especially designed to lull you into slumber
- If you habitually wake during the night, fretting about problems or with bright ideas, keep a pad by your bed and write them down
- When you wake up in the morning, make a decision to have a good day – that doesn't mean easy, but it does mean that you intend to go through the ups and downs in the best way possible

## ❧ 8

# Kitchen Medicine

Mankind survived for millennia by using food as medicine. Today, the use of common and garden (literally) ingredients is as relevant as ever for treating minor ailments in the family and workplace. You will almost certainly have these ingredients in your kitchen, or growing on your windowledge. We always recommend buying organic herbs and spices – like tea and coffee, these small plants are likely to be sprayed extensively with herbicides, as well as being artificially fertilised. If you're feeding your own homegrown herbs, use an organic preparation – unless you want a cocktail of synthetic chemicals with your herbal medicine. Always try to use fresh herbs, if possible.

---

### Grow your own herbal pharmacy

Many herbs are simple to grow. All you need is a few pots on a sunny windowsill; water them regularly and you have a natural pharmacy. Try mint, camomile, sage, feverfew, rosemary and thyme. Order from an organic source, if possible (see the Directory, pages 281 and 282). Many herbs do better with a light covering, to prevent attacks from opportunist insects. Fine

---

mesh, draped in a tent over the pot, will prevent the worst of the attacks. Your herbs are only as good as the soil in which they are grown, so change it from time to time, and offer plenty of good-quality organic fertiliser during the growing season.

You will see that there is also a small section on homeopathic remedies at the end of the chapter. We are firm devotees of homeopathy for all sorts of problems and to support conventional medicine, in the case of surgery, for instance.

As ever, the golden rule is that you should always consult a qualified health practitioner if any ailment continues for more than a couple of days, or gets worse.

**Anaemia: molasses and Marmite**
Pale lips and eye rims (on the inside) are the tell-tale signs of anaemia. Anaemia is often associated with fatigue and depression, rather than being simply a lack of iron in the bloodstream. To help anaemia you need a full spectrum of B vitamins plus vitamin C. The simplest old-fashioned kitchen remedy for anaemia is a combination of black-strap molasses and Marmite – but not together! Take about one dessert-spoonful of molasses and a teaspoon of Marmite daily. If the anaemia persists, you must see a healthcare professional because it may be a precursor of a more serious condition.

**Bad breath: drink water**
Dehydration increases body odour and bad breath, so the first thing to do is to make sure you are drinking enough water. The ideal is at least a litre of pure, still water, every day.

**Bad breath and mouth ulcers: rosemary and thyme mouthwash**

Put a sprig of fresh or dried rosemary and the same of thyme in a small teapot. Add boiling water and leave to stand for 10 minutes. When this is cool, use half as a mouthwash and drink the rest. This combination of these two herbs is a very effective antiseptic and can be used to help mouth ulcers as well. Drink 4 to 6 cups daily.

An instant remedy is to chew a few sprigs of parsley or mint.

**Bladder infections: cranberries**

One of the active ingredients in cranberries is hippuric acid, which raises the acidity of urine. That inhibits the spread and development of bacterial infections and stops the bacteria adhering to the urinary tract walls. Regular use of cranberries is also said to be beneficial for the kidneys and the heart. Sip about 10floz (300ml) cranberry juice throughout the day if you have a urinary tract infection. Avoid sweetened juices.

**Common cold or chill: cinnamon tea**

Cinnamon can help you perspire and is also a tonic, both of which are useful when you have a cold or chill. Put one teaspoon of powdered cinnamon, or a whole cinnamon stick, in a small teapot. Add boiling water and leave to stand for 10 minutes. Drink slowly when it has cooled enough to be comfortable. Drink 4 to 6 cups a day while symptoms last.

**Colds and coughs: garlic syrup**

Simply squeeze a few cloves, then cover with runny honey to draw out the garlic juices, which are powerful in every way. Suck this off a teaspoon about 4 times a day while symptoms last.

**Snuffly chest or sinus infections: ginger and garlic drink for tight chests and blocked-up noses**

Take a piece of peeled fresh ginger about the length and width of your thumb, and two peeled garlic cloves. Grate both into a small teapot, add boiling water and let it stand for 10 minutes before drinking slowly. You can make more simply by topping up with boiling water; the ginger gets stronger as it 'cooks'. If the taste is too strong, add honey. This potion frees the mucus so that you can clear a bad chest and blow a blocked-up nose. Drink 4 to 6 cups a day while symptoms last.

The grown-up version of this is honey, lemon, ginger and garlic posset with brandy. To a mug of hot but not boiling water, add one teaspoon of honey (preferably Manuka), the juice of a fresh lemon, a half- to one-inch (2.5cm) chunk of fresh ginger, chopped (or a pinch of dried ginger or cinnamon), a decent-sized clove of garlic crushed or chopped – and a dash of brandy if you wish. Drink 4 to 6 cups a day while symptoms last.

**Bad colds and flu, catarrh and fever: elderflower tea**

Infuse teabags or 1 teaspoonful of dried elderflowers in boiling water for about 10 minutes; drink 3 or 4 times daily. If you use loose elderflowers, don't forget to strain it!

**Flu that affects your digestion: elderflower and peppermint tea with yarrow**

This is good for flu that is affecting your digestion, giving you gastrointestinal symptoms, nausea or discomfort in your stomach. You can buy elderflower and peppermint teabags, or use dried herbs. Add a teaspoonful of dried yarrow (available at healthfood stores), a good general tonic, as you begin to recover. Drink 4 to 6 cups a day while symptoms last.

### Fever: chicken soup

The old adage counselling you to starve a fever is right because you want to unclog your digestion. Light, 'clean' food, such as organic chicken soup, vegetable broths and fresh fruit or vegetable juices are perfect.

### Sore throats: ginger lozenges

Suck chunks of crystallised ginger when your throat hurts, instead of a throat lozenge or cough sweet. You can also buy chunks of preserved ginger in honey, which are delicious, or simply put preserved ginger in runny honey yourself. Use the leftover honey to make honey and lemon drinks.

### Constipation: linseeds and lemon

This common condition varies with individuals. Some people feel constipated after missing a single bowel movement, others after a week. The most usual cause of constipation is poor diet. The best ongoing treatment for constipation is to follow your Biotype diet and correct any stress weaknesses. However, for the occasional bout of mild constipation, try this treatment. Soak a dessertspoon of linseeds in water overnight. In the morning, add a spoon of lemon juice and molasses, then drink the fluid and eat the seeds. You can also add linseeds to your morning juice (see page 174).

A popular Italian traditional remedy is to take a tablespoonful of olive oil twice a day, but do not try this if you have had your gall bladder removed.

### Diarrhoea: cinnamon, honey and salt

Chronic or persistent diarrhoea needs expert medical attention because it is very easy for a child or an adult to become dehydrated if diarrhoea is left untreated. Diarrhoea is usually caused by the body trying to purge itself of an unwanted substance, such as alcohol. For non-chronic and non-persistent diarrhoea, try this simple remedy. Simmer one teaspoonful of powdered cinnamon in still pure water for 20 minutes with half a teaspoonful of honey (preferably Manuka) and a pinch of salt. Allow to cool and then drink. This makes about two cupfuls that can be sipped over the course of half an hour.

If you don't have cinnamon, try Cayenne pepper, a fiery little herb that works wonders. Add a teaspoon of cayenne to a wineglass of warm still water, sweetened with half a teaspoonful of honey (preferably Manuka) and drink.

**Digestive discomfort: mint**
Mint is one of the oldest remedies for soothing indigestion of all kinds. Roman soldiers were advised to use it, according to one ancient herbal. It also relieves any nauseous headache after a fatty meal. Use fresh mint, if possible, or a herbal teabag if not. Either put a handful of torn fresh mint, stalks and all, in a teapot and stand for 10 minutes, then drink when cool. Or use a mint teabag as normal.

**Energising pick-me-up rosemary tea**
Infuse fresh (or dried) rosemary with boiling water for 10 minutes and drink in the morning as an energising pick-me-up if you're really exhausted.

**Headache: water, pears and bananas**
A significant number of headaches are due to dehydration or a drop in blood sugar levels. So before you hit the herbs or pills, do two things. First, sip a tall glass of warmish, still, pure water. Second, eat a ripe pear or banana. If the headache has

not improved in about 10 minutes, try chamomile tea if the headache is due to stress, or feverfew if it is more intense and migraine-like.

To make the tea, put one dessertspoonful of fresh or dried chamomile or feverfew, in a small teapot and fill with boiling water. Leave to stand then sip when at a drinkable temperature. Drink about two cupfuls.

Feverfew can be bitter, so add a teaspoon of honey to the infusion if you wish.

---

**Warning**

If you suffer from constant headaches, consult a qualified health professional immediately.

---

**Hiccups: fresh mint**

Hiccups may come from bolting your food without chewing it properly and/or swallowing air (see Chapter 4). Chewing your food thoroughly before swallowing and not eating on the run will help. If you get an attack, try our favourite treatment of chewing fresh mint. If you haven't got any fresh mint, go to the health store and get a herbal product that contains valerian. Granny's favourite tip of drinking from the wrong side of the class while holding both arms up in the air seems to work, too, but you have to be a contortionist to do it. And for the record, it also seems to work if you hold only one arm in the air – which is simpler.

## How to prevent coughs, colds and flu

Garlic is one of nature's medicinal power houses, due to a powerful chemical called allicin, which has an antibacterial, antiviral and anti-fungal effect. As with all medications that support the immune system, garlic should be used long term, as part of a lifestyle regime. Crushed over or in food is the simplest way.

This powerful plant, which again has been extensively researched, is excellent for warding off colds and coughs and keeping infections at bay generally. It also clears toxins from the gut, helping the digestion, and has been shown to be useful in reducing high blood pressure. It's better not to cook it too much, so add at the last moment to stir fries.

You can also make garlic tea by crushing three cloves and adding hot or boiling water. Leave to stand and sip when at a drinkable temperature. Drink one strong mugful at night (this avoids you breathing garlic over unrelated people; give your partner a mug too). If you are worried that your breath smells, chew a few sprigs of parsley.

You can also use garlic syrup for cold or coughs. Simply squeeze a few cloves, then cover with runny honey to draw out the garlic juices – powerful in every way.

### Preventing infection: hot spicy tea

A weak digestion is the perfect breeding ground for infection, according to Chinese medicine and herbalism. In the cold, damp of winter, we eat cold, damp food, such as wheat, milk and sugar, and we drink cold water. Instead, eat porridge sprinkled with cinnamon for breakfast, warming soups and stews for lunch and supper, and choose warm drinks such as this homemade 'yogi' tea.

Heat one pint (20floz/600ml) of pure water with 4 cloves, 4 black peppercorns, 4 cardamom pods, one cinnamon stick and some slices of fresh ginger. Simmer with the lid on for 15 to 20 minutes. Strain. This makes two large mugs: drink one mug twice daily.

### Mouth ulcers: sage tea

Mouth ulcers are very often associated with stress and a deficiency of nutrients in your body. If you are rundown and get ulcers, it is because you are depleted in vitamins C and B. If you are getting mouth ulcers regularly, take a vitamin B-complex product, plus 2 grams of vitamin C daily.

As well as the mouthwash for bad breath (see page 212), you can use a strong tea made of dry sage during a bout of mouth ulcers. Put three heaped teaspoons of sage in a small teapot, add boiling water and drink when cool enough. Use half as a mouthwash first, then drink the rest. You can also add rosemary and thyme (as above) to the sage tea.

### Nausea, travel sickness and morning sickness: ginger

Whether the nausea is from pregnancy, hangover, migraine or some form of transport, ginger is the universal treatment. In fact, NASA astronauts took it into space with them. Take a piece of ginger about the size of your thumb, peel, then chop or grate finely. Put in a small teapot, add boiling water and leave to stand for 10 minutes. Sip when at a drinkable temperature. You can top up this ginger with boiling water three or four times; each time it's used it becomes a little stronger. Ginger tea can also be drunk cold with crushed ice (made with pure water).

**Wind and flatulence: cinnamon, nutmeg and milk**

Add one teaspoonful of powdered cinnamon and a pinch of nutmeg to a glass of warm cow's milk or soya milk. Stir and drink for virtually instant relief.

**Wind and nausea: ginger tea**

Grate or chop a large chunk of peeled fresh ginger into a small teapot and add boiling water. Let it stand for 10 minutes and drink when comfortably warm. Top up with boiling water.

## Simple homeopathic remedies

Homeopathy is a simple, non-invasive way of helping your health holistically. To boost your wellbeing in the long term, you need to consult a naturopath or homeo-path for a personal prescription. But there are useful general remedies for immediate (acute) problems that are safe for family, friends and colleagues.

Homeopathic remedies don't work well with any strong-flavoured or -smelling substances, so avoid drinking coffee, brushing your teeth with a mint toothpaste, or using aromatherapy oils for at least 30 minutes either side of taking a remedy. Better still, choose a natural fennel, lemon or cinnamon toothpaste instead of your regular brand.

Take '6' potency remedies for everything outlined below, unless noted otherwise. This is the potency most commonly available in healthfood shops and chemists.

- *For runny nose, sneezing; cold sores; headaches after emotional upsets:* take Natrum mur, one twice a day until symptoms are relieved, up to a week

- *For colds with aches and pains, also recurrent fevers that you can't crack, lack of energy and sleepiness:* take Gelsemium, one twice a day for up to a week
- *For overindulgence in food, alcohol and cigarettes; headaches after eating too much; irritability linked with streaming cold and chills; overwork and late nights:* take Nux vomica, one twice a day for 3 or 4 days
- *For the mother who's had enough, and is depressed, fed up and wants – temporarily – to flee her family:* take Sepia, twice a day for up to a week
- *For sudden earache in children (while you wait for doctor) or for any sudden high temperature:* take Belladonna, every 3 hours, for up to 24 hours, then a cold remedy as above, if needed
- *For sudden flu-like feverish symptoms:* take Oscillo-coccinum 30, one every 3 to 5 hours for 24 hours
- *For waves of emotional trauma that threaten to overwhelm you (anything from office stress to disturbing world events to arguments with your partner):* take Ignatia, one tablet each time the emotional wave surfaces
- *For bumps and bruises:* take Arnica, one tablet immediately, another 30 minutes later, another the evening of the same day, and the fourth the next morning. Also have Arnica cream on hand to rub on children's (and grown-up's) sore bits
- *For insomnia:* take Carbo veg, 2 tablets at bedtime

## Dr Bach's Rescue Remedy

This blend of flower essences is invaluable for all traumas, physical, mental or emotional – big and small. It can safely be given to children of all ages, and even pets and plants. It also comes in liquid form (for internal or external use) and a cream for physical problems, including stings, sore skin, grazes, bites and itching.

# The Food File

We like food a lot. Much of the time we spent working on this book took place over various quite long meals. Roderick is a Pioneer and Sarah is a Hunter Gatherer so, in the main, we ate simple fish or meat and salad or vegetables that suited both our Biotypes beautifully. They also took very little time to prepare. For the sake of honesty, we have to confess that we quite frequently finished off the meals with our favourite sinful treat, Green & Black's Organic Chocolate or Organic Vanilla Ice-cream. (Fine on an occasional treat basis, according to Roderick.)

This chapter doesn't pretend to be a comprehensive recipe book, but it gives you some basic recipes and cooking techniques and ideas for mix and match dishes. There are also recipes and tips from some of Roderick's patients. In the Directory (see page 285), you will find our favourite recipe books. In this techno age, there is another wonderful source of recipes completely free: on the Net. For example, the Vegetarian Society provides a wealth of 'Cordon Vert' recipes and there are many other useful and inspirational websites. Again, these are included in the Directory.

## Feeding a family

Many families will have more than one Biotype repre-
sented and certainly when you entertain you are likely
to have several or all at the table. It may seem a mind-
boggling task to decide what to eat but take heart, it's
really quite simple. We absolutely don't suggest serving
different meals for each type. There are many combinations that will suit everyone.

Bear in mind that you will not be indentifying
Biotypes until after puberty, so children can eat the same
food as parents do. What they need most is good wholesome fresh food, preferably organic, and the minimum
of prepared food with additives.

If you look at the Biotypes again, you will see that
in many cases breakfast is the meal with most variations.
Many households already cater for different demands at
breakfast from eggs and bacon to muesli, via vegetarian
sausages and fruit soya yogurt, to toast and peanut butter.
Adults, and even most teenagers, can be left to prepare
their own breakfasts.

The simplest way to approach the midday and evening
meals is to serve dishes based on food combining, which
will suit everyone (see the section on Pioneers, pages
68–78). Protein (either animal or vegetarian) based
menus with vegetables and salads will suit everyone.

If you have vegetarians or vegans to feed, we suggest
you build the menu around vegetable and salad dishes,
then serve a vegetarian or vegan protein dish (see pages
90–95 for details of vegetarian/vegan requirements and
complete proteins), plus a simple animal/fish protein dish
such as roast chicken or baked fish.

Here are some suggestions for meals that will suit all the Biotypes; serve with green vegetables and salads, plus olive/garlic/coriander purée or tomato and basil sauce. (Also see the vegetarian section in Chapter 5.)

- Roast or poached chicken
- Roast or poached fish
- Quinoa risotto
- Quorn casserole with vegetables
- Tortilla/big thick flat omelette served warm or at room temperature
- Brown rice dish (hot or cold) with marinated carrot salad, and pineapple and cucumber salad
- Caesar salad with flaked almonds (not croutons), chopped fried bacon, chicken or tuna
- Avocado salad
- Vegetable stew with vegetarian protein (tofu, TVP, Quorn or vegetarian sausages)

---

**Tip**

If you're feeding a family, get in the habit of freezing individual portion of each person's favourite dish. Then, if there's a revolt about supper, you can haul it out immediately.

---

We're going to start by giving you basic recipe suggestions for dishes that can be eaten by all of the Biotypes. Some of you may be seasoned cooks, and these early recipes might be too simple for your tastes. However, many people have told us that they would eat more fish if they felt more confident about cooking it. Fish is very good for you (particularly oily fish) and you will see that it figures largely in the Biotype diets. Here are some basic cooking methods which we have found work simply and well.

---

### Herbs to flavour meat, poultry and fish

While you need to use leafy herbs in salads – to avoid spiky or rough textures, such as rosemary – you can use any and everything when you are using herbs for flavour. On the whole, fish lends itself to milder, sweeter herbs, such as parsley, mint, tarragon, chervil, while meat and poultry can support more robust tastes, such as rosemary, sage and thyme. These strong herbs make a marvellous bed on which to roast meat or chicken. Just experiment! The only potential troublespots are dried herbs because they have stronger, more concentrated flavours and they burn more easily – which is a problem if the herbs are mixed into a dish.

---

## Basic techniques for cooking fish

### Whole fish

- If you are going to cook a whole (or half) fish, such as salmon, to eat cold, the simplest, mistake-proof way is to use a big fish kettle, borrowed or bought.
- Lay the fish in the kettle, then fill with pure water, some white wine, as many mixed fresh sweet herbs as you can find, lots of salt and a few slices of lemon.
- Take the fish out and bring the flavoured water slowly to the boil, then simmer for about 10 minutes to make a well flavoured court bouillon.

- Put the fish in when the mixture is just off the boil.
- Turn off the heat, cover, put on a cool surface (tile or stone floor is excellent) and leave severely alone for several hours until the liquid is cool.
- Drain, skin, dress and serve with mayonnaise. Tart up bought mayo with lots and lots of chopped fresh herbs and lemon juice to taste, plus extra seasoning if you wish.

You can use exactly the same method if you want to serve the fish warm:

- Keep an eye on the fish and when the eye turns white and you can lift the skin easily off the flesh, take it out of the water.
- Proceed as before.
- Wear thin surgical gloves to skin the fish if you're serving it warm and eating with your guests, to avoid fishy bits under your nails and a fairly indelible (though temporary) pong.

### Fish Portions

There are two simple and speedy ways to cook fish portions: roasting 'naked' in a very hot oven or sealing in a foil or parchment envelope so that the fish steams as it bakes in a medium oven. The timings are approximate because they vary with different types and portion sizes of fish and different ovens. Comfortingly, it is very hard, if not impossible, to spoil the finished version unless you totally disregard these timings and overcook by a long way.

#### Roasting

Have your pieces of fish cut into 6 to 8oz (150–200g) portions. We use cod or salmon. Turn your oven to nearly maximum

– about 200°C, gas mark 7/8 or 500°F. The precise temperature really doesn't matter.

Lay your fish portions, skin side down, on an oiled baking sheet or in an ovenproof dish. Salt and pepper liberally.

Spread the top side with grainy mustard if you like. You can also add chopped herbs to the mustard.

Roast for about 10 minutes – the exact time will depend on your oven and the type of fish: salmon takes a few minutes longer than cod if the pieces are about the same size.

Test by putting a knife into the centre to see if it's done. If it's still raw, put back in the oven for a minute or two only.

Serve as soon as possible.

---

**Citrus dressing for meat, fish and poultry**

Serve plain meat, fish or poultry with lemon-flavoured olive oil (buy or make your own) in which you have put lots of chopped fresh herbs.

---

### Baking in an envelope

Again, have your pieces of fish cut into 6 to 8oz (150–200g) portions. Remember that flat thin pieces of fish, such as plaice or brill, will take a shorter time than thick-ish steaks or 'darnes' (pieces cut straight down the fish) of, say, halibut or turbot.

Lay on well-buttered pieces of foil or parchment about 10 inches (25cm) square – enough to fold up firmly but loosely around the fish so that it is completely encased.

Add a dessertspoonful of wine, the same of oil, or a knob of butter, some fresh herbs, plus salt and pepper; you can also put in a little grated fennel or onion, or other seasoning.

Bake in a preheated moderate oven, 180°C, gas mark 4, 350°F for 10 to 15 minutes.

## Sources of vegetarian and vegan protein

- Cheese
- Eggs
- Fish
- Tofu, all varieties (such as plain, smoked, flavoured, also soya meat in the form of TVP)
- Quorn
- Dried reconstituted beans of all kinds
- Lentils
- Chickpeas
- Quinoa
- Nuts: almonds, walnuts, hazelnuts, Brazil nuts, pine nuts
- Tahini (ground sesame paste)
- Mixed seeds: sunflower, pumpkin and sesame seeds

When you're substituting vegetable protein for animal sources, increase the serving by about 10 to 15 per cent. For instance, the average egg is about 35g in weight, about $1^1/3$oz.
In protein terms:

- 1 egg = $1^1/2$oz (40g) tofu
- 2oz (50g) hard cheese = $2^1/2$oz (65g) tofu
- 3oz (75g) fish = $3^1/2$oz (90g) tofu

## Main meals

### ੩ Mediterranean tofu casserole
Serves 4

1 packet tofu (about 8–10oz, 200–250g)
4oz (100g) aubergine, cut into $1/2$in/1cm dice

4 tbsp (60ml) olive oil

4oz (100g) onion chopped

7tbsp (100ml) garlic, crushed

1/2 mild green chilli, finely chopped

15oz (425g) tinned tomatoes, chopped

12floz (350ml) white wine

12floz (350ml) light vegetable stock or water

1 tbsp (15ml) tomato purée

2oz (50g) uncooked pasta (preferably spelt, rice or
    quinoa pasta)

4oz (100g) fennel, cut into 1/2-inch/1cm dice

4oz (100g) cauliflower, broken into small florets

4oz (100g) courgettes, cut into 1/2-inch/1cm dice

2oz (50g) broad beans

2oz (50g) pitted black olives, quartered

2 tbsp (30ml) mixed chopped fresh basil and thyme
    (or 1 tsp/5ml dried mixed herbs)

Sea salt and black pepper

Drain tofu, cut into 32 pieces. In a non-stick pan, fry tofu and aubergine gently in the oil, until evenly browned. Remove from pan. Add onion to the same pan and cook gently until softened. Add garlic and chilli and cook for a further minute. Add remaining ingredients, and the cooked tofu and aubergine. Simmer gently until pasta and vegetables are just cooked (about 7 minutes). Season to taste.

## ⋙ Smoked tofu paella
Serves 4

1 packet smoked tofu, (about 8–10oz, 200–250g), cut
    into 32 cubes/triangles

5 tbsp (75ml) olive oil

18oz (500g) mixed vegetables, cut into 1-in/2.5cm
   pieces (such as, peppers, baby sweetcorn, broccoli,
   mushrooms)

6oz (150g) onion, chopped

6oz (150g) carrot, cut into 1-in/2.5cm batons

2 tsp (10ml) garlic, crushed

1/2 mild green chilli, finely chopped

11oz (275g) brown rice

1 pint (20floz/600ml) white wine

1 pint (20floz/600ml light vegetable stock, double
   strength

6oz (150g) tomatoes, peeled and chopped

3oz (75g) pitted black olives, sliced

2 bay leaves

2 tbsp (30ml) chopped fresh tarragon (or 1 tsp/5ml
   dried)

1 tbsp (15ml) chopped fresh sage

2 tbsp (30ml) chopped parsley

Salt and black pepper

1 lemon, cut into 8 wedges

In a non-stick pan, fry tofu in oil over a medium heat until
light brown. Remove from pan. Increase heat and add the
mixed vegetables to the same pan. Cook until browned lightly.
Remove from pan. Place onions and carrots in same pan.
Cook gently until softened. Add the garlic, chilli and rice.
Cook for 1 minute. Add wine, stock, chopped tomatoes, olives
and bay leaves. Simmer, covered, until the rice is cooked
(about 25 minutes). Add more liquid, if necessary, during the
cooking time. Remove bay leaves. Add the tofu, vegetables
and fresh herbs. Season with salt, black pepper and lemon
juice. Garnish with lemon wedges.

## ≥**&** Californian style brochettes
Serves 4 as a snack, 8 as a starter (makes 8 x 12ins/30cm) skewers

> 1 packet tofu, (about 8–10oz, 200–250g) (try Cauldron
>     Original or Marinated), cut into 32 cubes
> 1 small pineapple, peeled and cut into 32 pieces
> 4oz (100g) large seedless black grapes
> 1 medium mango, peeled and cut into 12 pieces
> 4oz (100g) mango chutney
> 8 sprigs fresh herbs
> 1 lime, cut into 4 wedges

Thread skewers alternately with tofu, pineapple, grapes and mango. Brush with mango chutney. Cook under a pre-heated grill for 5 minutes until very hot and just browning. Serve immediately, scattered with fresh herbs, and garnished with wedges of lime.

## ≥**&** Mixed whole-grain salad with miso and tarragon dressing
Serves 4 to 6

This useful recipe, which is suitable for vegans as well as everyone else, comes from *The Detox Cook* (see the Directory, page 285).

> 2oz (50g) whole-wheatberries, soaked for 12 hours and
>     drained
> 2oz (50g) pot barley
> 2oz (50g) buckwheat groats
>
> *Dressing:*
> 2 tsp (10ml) brown miso

2 tsp (10ml) cider vinegar

2 tsp (10ml) soy sauce

1 tsp (5ml) olive oil

Bring a large pan of water to the boil and put in the grains (wheatberries and barley). Bring back to the boil and simmer for 50 to 60 minutes, until the grains are tender. Drain well and place in a bowl. Dry roast the buckwheat groats in a pan over a medium heat, until they give off a nutty aroma. Add plenty of water to cover, bring to the boil and simmer for 10 to 15 minutes, until tender. Drain well and add to the others. Mix together the dressing ingredients and stir into the hot grains so that the dressing is absorbed as the grains cool.

## ¿❧ Quinoa and cashew risotto

Serves 8

4 tbsp (60ml) olive oil

2 leeks, finely sliced

2 sticks celery, finely sliced

8 tbsp (120ml) quinoa

1 pint (600ml) water or white wine and water mixed

14oz (375g) tin water chestnuts

1oz (100g) cashew nuts

2 tbsp (30ml) sunflower seeds

Juice of 1 to 2 lemons

Sea salt and freshly ground black pepper

2 handfuls of fresh mint, chopped small

Heat the oil in a heavy pan and cook the celery and leeks till just soft. Add the quinoa and the liquid. Bring to the boil

and cook gently for 15 minutes, until the quinoa is soft and
has absorbed the liquid — add more if necessary. Drain the
water chestnuts and halve them, then add to the mixture.
Brown the nuts and sunflower seeds in a dry pan, then add
them to the risotto along with lemon juice, salt and pepper
to taste. Just before serving, stir in the fresh chopped mint.
Serve warm or cold.

### ‿ Beetroots and quinoa with red cabbage
Serves 6

16–20oz (400–500g) young beetroots, with their stalks
  and leaves
2 tbsp (30ml) olive oil
2 cloves garlic
1 medium leek
6oz (150g) quinoa
8oz (200g) red cabbage, finely sliced or chopped
16floz (500ml) water or vegetable stock
2oz (50g) pistachio nuts
3oz (75g) toasted cashew nuts
Sea salt and freshly ground black pepper

Remove stalks and leaves from the beetroots. Wash the beets.
Wash leaves, tear and set aside. Wash the stalks then chop
roughly. Steam the beetroots till nearly cooked then remove
from steamer and halve or quarter, depending on their size.
Meanwhile, heat the oil in a heavy-based pan, add the leeks
and garlic and cook gently for a few minutes. Add the quinoa,
red cabbage and liquid and bring to a simmer. Add the beetroots, plus stalks and leaves. Cover the pan and simmer gently
for 15 to 20 minutes, or until the quinoa has swelled and is

cooked. Most of the liquid should have been absorbed. Add the nuts, season to taste. Serve warm or at room temperature.

### ₰ Onions stuffed with sundried tomatoes, quinoa and anchovies
Serves 4

This recipe is dairy-, gluten- and egg-free, as well as being low-fat.

> 2 very large Spanish onions or 4 smaller ones
> 2 tbsp (30ml) olive oil
> 4 rashers bacon/bacon substitute, chopped small
> 1oz (25g) sundried tomatoes, plumped in boiling water
>   and then chopped, reserve the water
> 2oz (50g) mushrooms, chopped small
> 4oz (100g) fresh fennel, chopped small
> 4oz (100g) quinoa
> 1 tsp (5ml) dried or 1 tbsp (15ml) fresh basil leaves, torn
> 3½oz (100ml) white wine
> Water
> Sea salt and freshly ground black pepper

Slice off the top of the onions and enough of the root to allow them to stand up. Put in a dish and cook until the middles are partially cooked, try 10 minutes on high in a microwave or 20 to 30 minutes in a medium oven. Remove at least half of the onion from the middle using a knife and a spoon and chop roughly. Heat the oil in a heavy pan and add the partially cooked onion middles, the bacon rashers, tomatoes, mushrooms and fennel. Cook together gently for

3 to 4 minutes, then add the quinoa and basil and stir well. Make the tomato water up to 16floz (500ml) and add to the pot along with the wine. Bring all to the boil and simmer gently till the liquid is absorbed and the quinoa soft. Season to taste, then stuff as much as you can back into the hollowed-out onions. If you have used two big onions, cut them downwards in half to make four shells. Arrange them on a serving dish with the remaining filling around them and serve hot or at room temperature.

## ಀ Savoury lentil bake
Serves 4

> 2 medium onions, skinned and chopped
> 2 tbsp (30ml) olive oil
> 6oz (150g) lentils
> 1/2 tsp (2.5ml) dried basil
> 1/2 tsp (2.5ml) dried mixed herbs
> 2 tbsp (30ml) tomato purée
> 16oz (400g) can tomatoes
> 1 tsp (5ml) brown sugar
> Sea salt and freshly ground pepper

Soak lentils in plenty of water overnight. Add the herbs to the lentils and simmer until tender, according to directions on the packet. Fry the onions in the oil until soft. Add the drained lentils with all the other ingredients. Simmer for 15 minutes until thickened. Pour into ovenproof dish and bake at 180°C, gas mark 4, 375°F, for 20 minutes. Serve with crisp green salad.

## ‡⬤ Red hot rice

Serves 4

The recipe below is extremely spicy and it's not for the faint-hearted. You can, however, reduce the chilli and cayenne to taste, or omit them entirely.

  3 tbsp (45ml) olive oil

  1 large onion, finely chopped

  3 cloves garlic, crushed and chopped

  1 heaped tsp (5ml) ground cumin

  1 heaped tsp (5ml) ground coriander

  1 heaped tsp (5ml) ground paprika

  1 heaped tsp (5ml) ground turmeric

  1 tsp (5ml) chilli pepper, or leave out if preferred

  1 tsp (5ml) cayenne pepper, or leave out if preferred

  9oz (225g) basmati rice (washed and drained)

  10floz (300ml) skimmed milk

  1 tsp (5ml) sea salt, freshly ground black pepper

  9oz (225g) mange tout, topped and tailed, and halved

  4oz (100g) mushrooms, chopped

  4oz (100g) sultanas

  4oz (100g) currants, soaked

Heat oil in a large non-stick pan. Gently fry onions for two minutes, then add the garlic; cook until onions are translucent. Add the spices to the pan and cook for a further 5 minutes, stirring to make sure the mixture does not burn. Add the rice, stir and cook for a further 2 minutes. Add the milk, salt and pepper; stir, bring to the boil, cover and simmer for 15 to 20 minutes, until all the liquid has been absorbed. While the rice mixture is cooking, steam the mange tout and mushrooms with the fruit. When both mixtures are cooked, stir together and serve.

## Salads

These salads and vegetable dishes can be eaten on their own, as a starter or as a snack, or with protein (such as meat, fish, poultry, eggs, cheese and tofu) as part of a main course. They are appropriate for all of the Biotypes.

### Salad ingredients

Choose from any of these ingredients, especially those that are in season and locally produced. As with all food, always choose organic if possible. Better still, grow your own.

- Asparagus
- Avocado
- Baby broad beans
- Bean or seed sprouts
- Beans, all kinds
- Beetroot
- Broccoli florets
- Cabbage, white and red (sliced very thinly)
- Carrots (grated)
- Cauliflower florets
- Celery
- Chicory, white and red
- Chinese leaves
- Cucumber (peeled)
- Fennel
- Lettuce (all kinds)
- Mange tout
- Mushrooms
- Olives

- Peppers (red, orange, yellow or green bell or capsicums)
- Rocket
- Sorrel
- Spinach, baby
- Spring onions
- Tomatoes
- Watercress

Fruit:
- Grapes
- Grapefruit
- Orange
- Pears
- Pineapple

Fresh herbs:
- Basil
- Chervil
- Chives
- Coriander
- Marjoram
- Parsley
- Tarragon

Nuts:
- Toasted, flaked almonds or pine nuts
- Crumbled walnuts

## Crudités:

- French beans (not very fine)
- Broccoli or cauliflower florets

- Carrot or cucumber sticks
- Chicory leaves
- Peppers, cut in strips about a centimetre wide
- Spring onions
- Sugar snap peas

Serve with soya mayonnaise, humus, tzatziki (cucumber dip) or guacamole.

## ❧ Five-minute salad

**Serves 4**

1 large bag of mixed salad leaves, washed

*For the dressing:*
1 clove crushed garlic
4 tbsp (60ml) virgin olive oil
1 tbsp (15ml) balsamic vinegar
Lots of torn basil, tarragon and/or chervil
A little lemon juice
Sea salt and freshly ground black pepper to taste

*Optional extras:*
Edible flowers (such as nasturtiums)
Mixed bean sprouts
Chicory
Young spinach
Red leaves
Walnut pieces
Small pieces of orange section
Finely sliced fennel

Make dressing either in jar or in the bottom of a salad bowl. Put in salad. Toss at the last moment. Add any of the optional extras, as desired.

## ੨⬥ Basic spinach salad
Serves 4

Apply the same principles to other leaves and vegetables.

> 20oz (500g) baby spinach leaves, washed
> 8oz (200g) fine green beans, asparagus, cauliflower or
>    broccoli (or a mixture)
> About 8 sundried/sunkissed tomatoes, chopped
> 2oz (50g) of toasted sunflower seeds, crumbled walnut
>    pieces or toasted, flaked almonds

Put the spinach in a salad bowl. Prepare the beans (or other vegetable) by blanching, draining and cutting into small pieces. Add the beans and tomatoes to the bowl. Dress with enough of your favourite dressing to coat the vegetables lightly. Sprinkle on the sunflower seeds or nuts.

## ੨⬥ Basic mushroom salad
Serves 4

> 16oz (400g) small mushrooms
> Grated zest of 1 lemon
> 1 tbsp (15ml) of your favourite dressing, or walnut oil
> 1 tbsp (15ml) chopped parsley
> 1 tbsp (15ml) chopped capers

Slice the mushrooms finely and mix with parsley and capers.

Add lemon zest. Pour on the dressing, stir and chill for an hour before serving.

*Variation:*
Add fine green beans, sliced peppers, broccoli florets or chopped asparagus, or incorporate protein such as flaked tuna or cubed tofu.

## ੨ Marinated carrot salad
Serves 4

You can use the same dressing and procedure with virtually any hard vegetable, such as cauliflower, broccoli, asparagus and leeks.

    20oz (500g) carrots
    1 medium-size onion
    1 green pepper

    *Dressing:*
    3½floz (100ml) tomato juice
    3½floz (100ml) cider vinegar
    3½floz (100ml) virgin olive oil
    2 tsp (10ml) organic honey
    1 tsp (5ml) whole-grain mustard

Cut the carrots into matchsticks, place in a pan, cover with water, bring to the boil and allow to simmer for 4 to 5 minutes, until just tender. Drain and cool. Slice the onion into fine rings. Slice pepper finely, and remove the seeds. Mix the carrots with the onions and pepper. Mix dressing ingredients and marinade the vegetables in the dressing overnight.

## ?&. Cauliflower salad
Serves 4

> 1 small cauliflower head
> 2oz (50g) walnut pieces (small)
> 2oz (50g) finely chopped apricots
> 1 sliced and seeded pepper
> Grated rind and juice of 1 small orange
> Chopped parsley or coriander (optional)

Cut the cauliflower into tiny florets and finely grate the stalk. Put in a bowl, and add pepper, walnuts and apricots. Stir, then add orange juice. Season with sea salt and freshly ground pepper. Garnish with parsley or coriander, if you wish.

## ?&. Mange tout and avocado salad
Serves 4 to 6

> 16oz (400g) young mange tout, top and tail and remove
>     strings if necessary, or fine green beans
> 2 small/medium avocados, peeled and chopped small
> 2oz (50g) small fresh mushrooms, finely chopped
> 2 tbsp (30ml) olive oil
> 1 tbsp (15ml) lemon juice
> Sea salt and freshly ground black pepper
> 2 tbsp (30ml) parsley, finely chopped

If the mange tout (or beans) are very young and tender, just top and tail them and use raw in the salad. If a little older, boil them for 2 to 3 minutes. Combine the mange tout (or beans), avocados, mushrooms, olive oil, lemon juice, salt and black pepper and toss them well together. Garnish with parsley and serve.

## 🐸 Radicchio salad
Serves 4

1 large head radicchio
4 medium-sized tomatoes
1 peeled red onion
4oz (100g) radishes
1 sliced red pepper
3 tbsp (45ml) tomato juice
1 tbsp (15ml) balsamic vinegar
2 tsp (10ml) of virgin olive oil
A few leaves of sage, finely chopped or torn

Tear the radicchio into bite-sized pieces. Put in a salad bowl. Finely chop the onions. Skin and deseed the tomatoes, chop flesh, and mix with onions. Add to the bowl. Slice radishes and peppers finely. Add to the bowl. Blend tomato juice with virgin olive oil, vinegar and chopped sage, and pour over salad. Toss lightly just before serving.

## 🐸 Cucumber and spring onion salad
Serves 6

3 cucumbers, peeled if skin is bitter or thick, sliced thinly
4 spring onions, thinly sliced crossways
1 tbsp (15ml) fresh mint, finely chopped
1 small cup (about 250ml) natural yoghurt
Fresh mint to garnish

Lay the sliced cucumbers in a dish for an hour or so with a plate on top, until the liquid starts seeping out. Mix this with the yoghurt and mint, season to taste. Add the onions to the cucumbers and stir in the yoghurt mixture. Garnish with fresh mint.

*Variation:*

You can also use these quantities to make a cold cucumber soup: simply grate the peeled cucumbers, chop the spring onions very finely and add the other ingredients. Leave to stand and thin with still water to soup consistency, if necessary.

## ๕ Chinese cabbage and spinach with pomegranate and poppy seed dressing
Serves 4

> ½ largish Chinese cabbage (about 16oz/400g), thinly sliced crosswise
> 4oz (100g) young spinach leaves, washed, drained and chopped
> 1 pomegranate

> *Dressing:*
> 4floz (100ml) sunflower or other vegetable oil
> 2 tbsp (30ml) lemon juice
> 1 tsp (5ml) poppy seeds
> 1 tsp (5ml) cider vinegar
> 1 tsp (5ml) honey

Combine the Chinese cabbage and spinach leaves in a bowl. Cut the pomegranate and break out the seeds into the bowl with a small fork or teaspoon, avoiding adding any of the bitter yellow skin. Blend the dressing ingredients together until smooth and pour over the ingredients in the bowl. Don't add it all at once: you don't want to drown the salad, just coat the leaves. Toss well, turn the salad into a serving bowl and serve.

### 🐌 Mushroom salad with celery or fennel
Serves 4

> 3 large mushrooms or a small box of mixed field and
>   woodland mushrooms, washed and finely sliced
> 2 sticks celery, finely sliced *or* 1 large fennel bulb
> 1oz (25g) of soaked almonds and walnuts, chopped
> 1 medium-sized sweet crunchy apple, diced (core but
>   don't peel)
> 1 bunch watercress, torn into sprigs
>
> *Dressing:*
> 1 dsp (20ml) mayonnaise
> 3 dsp (60ml) natural yoghurt
> 1 tsp (5ml) whole-grain mustard
> Sea salt and freshly ground black pepper

Put watercress round large dish. Mix ingredients for dressing and season to taste. Put salad ingredients in bowl, pour over dressing and mix lightly. Spoon salad on to a plate and serve.

### 🐌 Carrot and redcurrant salad
Serves 4

> 16oz (400g) carrots, scrubbed and coarsely grated
> 4oz (100mg) redcurrants, removed from their stalks
> 1 tbsp (15ml) redcurrant jelly
> 2 tbsp (30ml) lemon juice

Combine the carrots and redcurrants and mix well together. Stir the redcurrant jelly into the lemon juice. Toss the salad in this mixture, then set it aside in the refrigerator to chill before serving.

## ?❧ Fennel and grapefruit salad

Serves 4

> 16oz (400g) bulb fennel, washed and trimmed
> 2 grapefruits, peeled and pith cut away, and separated
>    into segments with a sharp knife, then halved
> 2 tbsp (30ml) olive oil
> 1/2 tsp salt
> A few fennel leaf sprouts for garnishing

Cut and throw away the hard cores of the fennel bulbs. Slice the bulbs into thin sections and place these in a salad bowl. Prepare the grapefruit segments with a sharp knife over the bowl, letting the chunks fall over the fennel. Add the olive oil and the salt and mix thoroughly. Garnish with the fennel leaves and serve.

## ?❧ Pear, grape and cucumber salad

Serves 4 to 6

> 3 ripe but firm sweet pears, peeled, cored; one pear
>    thinly sliced, the rest diced
> 1/2 medium cucumber, divided in half lengthways, seeds
>    scooped out. Slice half of the cucumber, dice the rest
> 4oz (100g) black or green seeded or seedless grapes,
> Vinaigrette dressing (to taste)

Make a bed of the pear and cucumber slices in a small salad bowl. Put the remaining pear, cucumber and grapes (reserve 5 or 6 grapes) into a bowl and toss them in vinaigrette dressing to taste. Pour this mixture over the bed of pear and cucumber slices. Garnish the salad with the reserved grapes, chill and serve.

## 🐌 Caribbean salad
Serves 4

4-in/10cm piece of cucumber, quartered lengthways and
   chopped crosswise
2 medium just-ripe bananas, thinly sliced
2 medium green peppers, seeded, cored and diced
2 sweet oranges, peeled, pith removed, separated into
   segments and then cut into halves
5floz (150ml) natural yoghurt
1 tbsp (15ml) flaked almonds, lightly toasted

Combine the cucumber, banana, green pepper and oranges
in a salad bowl. Stir in the yoghurt, sprinkle the almonds over
the top and serve.

## 🐌 Pineapple and cucumber salad
Serves 4

Tinned pineapple is acceptable as long as it is not tinned in
sugar, or with syrup.

6oz (150g) pineapple, fresh or tinned, cut into small
   chunks
1 large cucumber, peeled and sliced thinly
1 red pepper, sliced and deseeded
1 tsp (5ml) finely chopped fresh mint
2 dsp (60ml) finely chopped dried fruit, such as apricots,
   sultanas and figs
1 dsp (20ml) toasted sesame seeds

Soak the dried fruit in a little pineapple juice for at least 30
minutes. Mix the pepper, pineapple and soaked dried fruit

together. Lay the sliced cucumber overlapping on a dish or plate. Put the mixture on top. Sprinkle sesame seeds over the top, and serve.

## A meal in a salad

### ?❧ Gado-gado
Serves 4

Gado-gado is a popular Indonesian dish consisting of a mixture of raw and cooked vegetables arranged on a serving dish and served with a spicy peanut sauce, either poured over them or in a side bowl. It is light, crunchy, tasty and healthy. The vegetables suggested in the ingredients list may be changed to suit availability or personal preference. If you do not like moderately hot food, omit the chilli in the sauce or use less than suggested.

> 1/2 medium cucumber, sliced
> 4oz (100g) beansprouts, washed and drained
> 1/2 crisp head lettuce, washed and torn
> 2 medium potatoes, peeled and chopped
> 4oz (100g) French beans, top, tail and stringed, cut into
>     2-in (5cm) lengths
> 2 medium carrots, peeled, cut in half and then thickly
>     sliced lengthways
>
> *Sauce:*
> 1 tbsp (15ml) vegetable oil
> 1 clove garlic, crushed
> 1/2 medium onion, finely diced
> 1/2 red chilli, seeds removed, chopped or 1/4 tsp hot
>     pepper sauce

4oz (100g) peanut butter
2 tsp (10ml) brown sugar
2 tsp (10ml) lemon juice
8floz (240ml) coconut milk (or water)
Salt to taste
1 hard-boiled egg, sliced, as garnish

To make the sauce:
Heat the oil in a small pan and sauté the garlic, onion and chilli pepper until softened. Put the contents of the pan into a blender and add the peanut butter, sugar, lemon juice and water. Process to a smooth sauce and then pour the sauce back into the pan. Bring the sauce to a gentle boil with occasional stirring, salt to taste and set on a low simmer.

To make the salad:
Put the potatoes on to boil and cook until just tender. Boil the carrots and beans in salted water to just cover, for 5 minutes only, drain. Arrange the cucumber, beansprouts, lettuce, cooked potatoes and lightly cooked French beans and carrots in a serving dish. Garnish with slices of hard-boiled egg and serve with the hot peanut sauce poured over or in a separate bowl.

## ❧ Tahini, nut and vegetable rice salad
Serves 4

This is a good filling meal on its own, great to take to work or on picnics.

16oz (400g) cooked long grain brown rice
4oz (100g) red cabbage, finely chopped or grated
1 small green pepper, seeded, thinly sliced and chopped

1 small carrot, scrubbed and grated

1oz (25g) sultanas

1oz (25g) cashew nut pieces

2floz (60ml) tahini (sesame paste)

2floz (60ml) yoghurt

1 tbsp (15ml) lemon juice

Sea salt and black pepper to taste

Combine the rice with the red cabbage, green pepper, carrot, sultanas and cashew nuts. Combine the tahini, yoghurt and lemon juice. Season to taste with sea salt and black pepper. Pour the dressing over the salad and mix well.

## ≥♣ Brown rice salad

Serves 4

This is a simple brown rice salad, where the rice is cooked and marinated in vinaigrette with herbs. It is a good staple and can be used with all the different kinds of grains, such as wild rice (which is, in fact, a grass seed), rye, spelt, cous cous, sweetcorn and barley, either singly or mixed.

8oz (200g) brown rice, rinsed twice in cold water to
    remove excess starch and dust

20floz (500ml) water

*Dressing:*

4 tbsp (60ml) olive oil

2 tbsp (30ml) white wine/cider vinegar

1 clove garlic, crushed

2 tbsp (30ml) fresh chives and parsley (and/or other
    herbs), finely chopped

Sea salt and freshly ground black pepper

Bring the water to boil and add the brown rice (you don't need to add salt at this point because the dressing adds the flavour). Stir, then cover and cook gently for 20 to 30 minutes until the rice is soft and virtually all the water has been absorbed. While the rice is cooking, mix the dressing ingredients together. Add to the rice while hot or warm. The rice will then absorb all the dressing. Arrange in a bowl, and serve.

### ⅔ Smoked tofu salad with broccoli, mushrooms, sweetcorn and pineapple
Serves 4

This high protein salad is suitable for all types, but especially the Farmer Gardener and the Dancer type.

> 1 packet smoked tofu, (about 8–10oz, 200–250g) cut
>    into ¹/₂-in (1cm) cubes
> 8oz (200g) of broccoli florets
> 4oz (100g) mushrooms, wiped clean and thinly sliced
> 4oz (100g) pineapple or orange, in small pieces about
>    the same size as the tofu
> 1 dsp (20ml) frozen sweetcorn
> Sea salt and freshly ground black pepper
> Herbs such as parsley, coriander, mint, basil, chopped or
>    torn
> Your favourite dressing

Blanch the broccoli for 2 to 3 minutes, then cool. Put all ingredients in a dish or bowl. Dress with a little vinaigrette, walnut oil and lemon juice, to coat. Mix the ingredients gently, including all but one dessertspoon of herbs. Check seasoning. Garnish with the remaining herbs.

## Dressing

### 𝑒𝐿 Vinaigrette dressing

**Makes 5floz (150ml). Keep in the refrigerator.**

4floz (120ml) cold-pressed, extra virgin olive (or other
   vegetable) oil
2 tbsp (30ml) wine vinegar, cider vinegar or lemon juice
Salt and pepper to taste
1 tsp (5ml) prepared mild mustard (optional)
Extras: herbs, garlic, lemon juice, runny honey

Place all ingredients in a bowl or liquidiser and beat or blend
well. Test and adjust seasoning if necessary.

### 𝑒𝐿 Soya garlic mayonnaise

**This makes a standard jam jar full. Keep in the refrigerator.**

1 packet silken tofu (8–10oz, 200–250g) (ordinary if you
   can't find silken)
4 dsp (80ml) olive oil
1 dsp (20ml) balsamic vinegar
2 cloves garlic (more if you like it stronger)
1/2 tsp (2.5ml) whole-grain mustard
1/2 tsp (2.5ml) dill seed

Blend all ingredients until smooth and use as ordinary mayonnaise. Add herbs if wished.

### ❧ Olive purée with garlic and coriander
**Makes enough for 4 to 6**

This is wonderful with fish, meat, poultry or hot vegetables. Also as a spread on fresh bread, topped with tomatoes.

> 1 small jar or tub of black olive paste or purée (you can
> also find this as freshly-made tapenade in deli-
> catessens, or you can make it yourself by putting
> pitted black olives into a blender or food processor)
> 4 to 6 fat cloves garlic
> 1 bunch coriander, leaves

Roast the garlic in a hot oven until soft, then squeeze out the pulp. Wash the coriander and de-stalk. In a food processor, or with a pestle and mortar, or big wooden spoon and bowl, combine the black olive purée with the garlic pulp and coriander leaves. If you are not using a food processor or blender with a cutting blade, chop the coriander very finely. Decant into a bowl or jar and serve.

---

### Make your own superfoods: sprouted beans, seeds or grains

Most people remember sprouting mustard and cress seeds as a child. All that was required were some seeds and a piece of blotting paper, which you kept damp. You can use exactly the same principle to sprout your own beans, seeds or grains.

All you need is a big wide-mouthed jar (such as a Kilner jar) and some dried beans, wholegrains or seeds, which you can buy in a healthfood store. You can sprout pretty well any of these

---

that are suitable for eating. A mixture of mung beans, wheat grains and alfalfa seeds are a popular choice.

- Place the seeds, beans or grains in the bottom of the jar. You will need to lay them about $1/2$ in (10mm) deep, to make enough for one serving.
- Cover the mouth of your sprouting jar with muslin, cheese-cloth or nylon mesh and secure with a rubber band over and around the top.
- Pour filtered water into the jar through the muslin until it covers the seeds, and gently swirl the jar so that the seeds are soaked. Then turn the jar upside down to remove excess water. Do this twice.
- This will leave you with a damp pile of seeds in the jar, which are just moist enough to start sprouting.
- Stand the jar upside down to remove excess water.
- Leave the jar on its side in the shade at living-room temperature.
- Repeat the wetting process above two or three times a day.
- By the end of the second day, you should have a crop of sprouts.
- Take them out of the jar and put in a bowl of water. The outer husks will just float off.
- Strain and your own spanking fresh sprouts are ready to use in a salad, or as you wish.

---

## Useful snacks for all types

- Crudités (see page 238)
- Avocado pear
- Fruit
- Nuts: almonds, hazelnuts, Brazils or pine nuts
- Mixed nuts and raisins
- Sunflower or pumpkin seeds

---

## Super sandwich for all types

- Wholegrain or rye bread
- Sliced avocado (sprinkled with lemon if for picnic) or guacamole

Plus:
- Any green salad leaves, including baby spinach and rocket
- Black olive paste (if liked)
- Sundried or sunblush tomatoes, chopped or sliced
- Pine nuts

---

## Hot vegetable dishes

### ૨ Ratatouille
Serves 4

This French vegetable stew, said to have come from a gypsy recipe, can be eaten on its own or served with meat, poultry, some fish (not the delicate-flavoured types; cod is a good choice), pasta, tofu, quorn, cracked wheat, rice, lentils and chickpeas.

2oz (50g) finely chopped onion

2 cloves garlic, crushed

2 tablespoons (30ml) olive oil

20oz (500g) courgettes (or marrow)

20oz (500g) tomatoes, skinned, deseeded and chopped

1 red pepper, roasted, skinned, deseeded and roughly
  chopped

1 tbsp (15ml) parsley, chopped

Sea salt and freshly ground pepper to taste.

Cook garlic and onions slowly with the olive oil in a heavy pan for about 10 to 15 minutes until translucent. Add the remaining ingredients and simmer for about 20 to 30 minutes until the vegetables are tender: do not overcook to a mushy brown pulp. Serve hot or at room temperature with plenty of torn or chopped fresh parsley or basil on top.

## 𝆕 Oven-roasted vegetables

Serves as many as you like!

This is so simple you really don't need a recipe.

*Try these vegetables:*

Peppers, red, yellow, orange (green doesn't taste nice) –
  slice into 6 to 8 long segments and deseed

Tomatoes – use whole, cut a cross in the top

Asparagus – trim woody base and use whole

Big mushrooms – wipe clean, remove stalk and drizzle
  with oil

Courgettes – top and tail, slice lengthways into quarters

Small onions – trim top and bottom and bake in their
  skins

You can also use leaf vegetables, such as chicory, red
and white, and radicchio, but you must keep them
whole, or the leaves will burn; paint them well with
olive oil

Heat your oven until it's very hot. In a big roasting tin, lay
a selection of non-root vegetables cut into roughly equal sizes.
This is a peasant Mediterranean dish so don't be itty bitty.
Drizzle them with oil, season with sea salt and ground black
pepper. You can strew on some rosemary branches, if you like.
Take them off when the vegetables are cooked. Don't use
dried rosemary because it tastes nasty when roasted, and fishing
the bits out is a nightmare. Roast until the vegetables are
biteable-soft and taste sweet. Check after 15 minutes. Serve
warm or at room temperature with more olive oil, and
parmesan shavings (use a potato peeler).

## 🐾 Paul's root vegetable stew for Pioneers, Farmer Gardeners and Dancers
Serves about 4

3 medium carrots, peeled and sliced

1 large onion, finely chopped

1 clove garlic, finely chopped

1 small swede, peeled and chopped into 1/2 inch dice

1 small turnip, peeled and chopped into 1/2 inch dice

1 stick celery, washed and sliced

2 dsp (40ml) olive oil

1 large glass red wine

1 pint (20floz/500ml) vegetable stock (homemade or use
2 stock cubes)

Warm the olive oil in a large pan. Add the onions and garlic and fry until translucent. Add the vegetable stock and bring to the boil. Add the chopped vegetables and the red wine. Simmer until the vegetables are cooked and you have a dense stew (about half an hour). Serve with ready-prepared vegetarian dumplings or sausages, brown rice or any other grain.

## Steamed vegetables

It's worth investing in a vegetable steamer, which are widely available. Steaming vegetables is probably the most economic and nutritious way to cook vegetables. Steaming takes less time, cooks at a hotter temperature than boiling and you don't dunk the vegetables in the water, so steamed veggies retain more vitamins and minerals.

## ୧୬ Three vegetable mix
Serves as many as you want

> Carrots, broccoli and cauliflower or any other combination of seasonal vegetables
> Olive oil
> Sea salt and black pepper to taste
> Torn fresh herbs (optional)

Scrub the carrots and cut the cauliflower and broccoli into florets; cut the stalks into small cubes or slices. The finer you cut the vegetables the quicker they cook. Steam for about 10 minutes. Serve in a warmed dish and drizzle on a little virgin olive oil. Season to taste, and add torn fresh herbs if you like.

# Fruit puddings

## ੬ Fruit fool
Serves 4

> 8oz (200g) fresh berries or other soft fruit, such as apri-
>     cots, rhubarb or gooseberries
> 2 tbsp (30ml) clear honey
> 4oz (100g) Greek yoghurt
> A few toasted almonds or hazelnuts

Rinse fruit and stew with a very little water until softened.
Drain any excess liquid. Add honey and leave to cool. When
cool, fold in yoghurt, put in individual glasses and chill.
Garnish with nuts and serve.

## ੬ Baked apples with fruit
Serves 3

> 2 tbsp (30ml) concentrated apple or pear juice
> 4 tbsp (60ml) water
> 2 tbsp (30ml) honey
> 1 tbsp (15ml) mixed spices
> 3 baking apples
> 8oz (200g) dried fruit
> Yoghurt or fromage frais to serve (optional)

Put the concentrated juice, water, honey and mixed spice into
a large bowl and mix well. Wash and core apples. Fill with
the dried fruit. Pour liquid mixture over top. Place apples in
an oven dish and bake for 35 to 45 minutes at 200°C, gas
mark 6, 400°F. Serve with yoghurt or fromage frais.

## &✿ Fruit dream

**Serves 4 to 6**

> 16oz (400g) fresh soft berries
> 10oz (250g) silken tofu (you can use ordinary tofu but it
>    won't produce as fine a result)
> Juice of $1/2$ lemon
> 2 tbsp (30ml) runny honey
> A few drops of pure vanilla essence (not vanilla
>    flavouring)

Wash and hull fruit, leaving a few aside for decoration. Drain tofu and put into a liquidiser together with fruit, lemon juice and honey. Liquidise until smooth; add vanilla essence to taste and mix well. Divide into individual glasses or small bowls, chill until required. Serve decorated with remaining fruit.

## &✿ Fruity rice pudding

**Serves 4**

> 1 can ready-made organic rice pudding
> 8oz (200g) of dried dates, figs and pears
> 1oz (25g) flaked almonds, toasted

Chop the dried fruit finely and mix with rice pudding. Serve hot or cold, garnished with toasted almonds.

## Basic recipes

### Breakfast

### ›❧ Original bircher muesli
Serves 1

Muesli is best prepared the night before. Soaking the grains and leaving them to stand in the refrigerator over night softens the fibre content and reduces the impact on the digestive tract. It also begins to liberate essential nutrients from the food. People with IBS-type problems may find this type of muesli is easier to cope with.

Any grain mix can be treated in this way. Softened grains can be eaten with dried fruit and yoghurt for breakfast or as a dessert. If you don't like yoghurt, swap it with fruit juice (apple or grape). For dessert, it tastes divine made with cranberry juice.

>  2 to 3 small apples, 1 large or 2 small pears, or their
>     dried fruit equivalent
>  1 tbsp (15ml) walnuts, hazelnuts or peeled almonds
>  1 level tbsp (15ml) porridge oats
>  1 tsp (5ml) runny honey
>  1 dsp (20ml) full-cream milk or soya milk
>  Juice of ½ lemon

Mix oats with honey and milk. Grate the apples (skin, core and pips) into a separate bowl and add the lemon juice, then stir into the oats. Add the nuts. Then leave overnight.

## ❧ Rod's muesli and nut porridge
Serves 1

> ½ cup (125ml) of muesli base from a healthfood store
> 2 tsp (10ml) cracked linseeds
> 1 dsp (20ml) sunflower seeds, pumpkin seeds and
>    sesame seeds
> Also add: broken or flaked almonds, walnuts, hazelnuts,
>    and/or pecans, chopped dried apricots, flaked
>    coconut, as you wish

Combine the night before. Place in a bowl and add milk or fruit juice to cover generously. Put a small plate on top with a weight. In the morning, the nuts, grains and seeds will have softened and expanded to make a gorgeous, soft, high-protein muesli. If it's a cold day, heat the muesli quickly to make a porridge. Put a little runny honey on top, with yoghurt if you like, for a totally scrummy dish.

## ❧ Breakfast summer pudding
Serves 4

All types can eat this as a delicious breakfast occasionally. It's also a great picnic pud.

> 4 to 6 slices thinly sliced wholemeal bread, crusts cut off
> 4oz (100g) strawberries
> 4oz (100g) raspberries
> 4oz (100g) blackberries
> (or any mixture of similar fruits)
> Yoghurt or fromage frais to serve (optional)

Wash the fruit gently but thoroughly. Take a medium-sized

pudding bowl and line with the bread, cut to fit and slightly overlapping at the joins. Don't omit the base. Leave one slice of bread as a lid. Take 2oz (50g) of each fruit and purée separately. Place a layer of halved strawberries in the bread-lined bowl and spoon on a little strawberry purée. Do the same with each of the fruits and purées, until all are used up. It should be very juicy so that the bread will become soaked. Take the remaining bread and make a lid to cover the fruit in the lined bowl. Take a small plate or saucer, place on top of the lid. Weight down with old-fashioned weights, or cans, to form a press. Chill overnight. Turn out and serve with yoghurt or fromage frais.

## ❧ Fruit breakfast muffins

**Makes 10**

> 4oz (100g) spelt or gluten-free flour
>
> 2 tsp (10ml) baking powder
>
> 3oz (75g) bran
>
> 4oz (100g) chopped apricots, figs or other dried fruit
>
> 1 dsp (20ml) molasses
>
> 10floz (300ml) skimmed milk
>
> 1 small egg
>
> 3 tbsp (45ml) safflower oil (you can use olive oil, but
>     choose a very light one)

Sieve flour and baking powder into a bowl. Stir in bran and chopped fruit. Mix molasses, milk and egg well together and pour into bowl of flour and fruit. Stir well and divide into 10 well-oiled muffin tins. Bake for about 25 minutes at 200°C, gas mark 6, 400°F.

## Barbara's sugar-free treats

These no-sugar recipes came from Barbara Symes, a patient of Roderick's.

### 🐾 Sugar-free gooey flapjacks

> 20oz (500g) porridge oats
> 4oz (100g) chopped dried apricots or sultanas
> 9oz (225g) unsalted butter, melted
> 1/3 bottle (7–10floz/210–300ml) concentrated apple or
>     pear juice (we use Meridian concentrate)

In a big bowl, mix together the oats, dried fruit and melted butter. Add the concentrated apple or pear juice until you have sticky but not sloppy mixture. Put into a non-stick or oiled tin. We use a square baking tin, about 3 inches (7.5cm) deep, and 10 by 10 inches (25 by 25cm). Put in a medium oven (about 180°C, gas mark 5, 350°F), and check after 15 to 20 minutes. When the mixture starts to go brown all over, take it out. Cut through into small portions – these are very filling. Leave in the tin until cool: the flapjacks will solidify.

### 🐾 No-sugar carob mousse
Serves 4

> 4oz (100g) cashew nuts or 4oz (100g) soaked peeled
>     almonds
> 1 to 2 ripe bananas
> 1 heaped tbsp (15ml) carob powder
> 4–5floz (120–150ml) soya milk or soya cream

Put the nuts into a food processor and reduce to fine-ish powder. Add the bananas and carob and process gently until mixed. Add soya milk until the mixture is light but not too sloppy. Pour into glasses or small coffee cups. Chill for 90 minutes, then serve.

### ❧ Ruffles

**Makes about 30**

This is a high-protein and no-sugar hit, which is invaluable for journeys.

> 4oz (100g) sesame seeds, toasted hazel nuts (shaken
>     in sieve to remove skins) and skinned almonds
> 4oz (100g) dates and raisins
> 2 tbsp (30ml) sugar-free peanut butter
> 2 tbsp (30ml) barley malt extract
> Carob powder to coat

Put the nuts and dried fruit in a food processor and whiz until you have a fine, smooth-ish mixture. Add the peanut butter and the barley malt extract and process until you have a ball-like pastry dough. Take it out, make small balls like truffles, and roll in carob powder.

## Bread

This recipe comes from Caroline Wilson, whose husband David manages the Prince of Wales' farm at Highgrove in Gloucestershire. It is a simple method of making delicious bread. The most important thing is to get the liquid the right temperature, too hot and the bread will be heavy. You can use different sorts of flour but you may need to use slightly less or more liquid, so don't slosh it all in at once. A convenient place to 'prove' the dough is to put it in a big covered dish in a very low oven with the door open. When you prove the loaves in their tins, cover with a dishcloth.

### ॐ Duchy Home Farm Organic Bread Recipe

> 1.5 kg organic wholemeal flour, Maris Widgeon from
> Shipton Mill if possible
> (You can substitute The Stamp Collection's Wheat-Free
> All-Purpose Flour, or you can make up a mixture of
> the Stamp Collection flour and rye flour, which is
> delicious.)
> 2 sachets dried yeast
> 1 tbsp (15ml) fine sea salt
> 1 tbsp (15ml) runny honey
> 6 tbsp (15ml) sunflower and/or olive oil
> 1 and 3/4 pints warm water (35floz/1050ml): this needs
> to be the tepid side of warm, so water you would
> bath a baby in
> Herbs, sliced olives, chopped sundried tomatoes, sultanas
> and nuts can be added to this basic recipe, as you wish

Combine flour and yeast in big mixing bowl. Dissolve honey and salt in a tea cup of warm water from the water above. Add oil and make up to 2 pints (40floz;1200ml) with warm water. Add liquid to flour and mix. Turn out onto a floured surface and knead until the dough is smooth, springy and alive. Leave covered to rise until doubled in size. Knead down again and divide into three oiled two-pound (32oz/800g) loaf tins. Preheat oven to 240°C, gas mark 8, 450°F). Cover loaf tins and leave to rise until nearly double size. Bake for 35 minutes, take out and tap bottoms of loaves – if they sound hollow, put loaves to cool on wire tray. If not, replace in oven for 5 minutes.

## Extras

### 𝄞 Hummus

Serves 2 to 3, or more as part of mixed dips

> 1 14oz (400g) can chickpeas, drained and rinsed
> Juice of a lemon
> 4 tbsp (60ml) olive oil
> 2 tbsp (30ml) light tahini
> 1 clove garlic, crushed
> 2 tbsp (30ml) pure water
> Sea salt and freshly ground pepper, to taste

Blend or process all ingredients together. Store in refrigerator. Serve with crudités.

---

### Guilt-free drinks

#### 𝄞 Pink fizz

Serves 1

> Water melon has the highest concentration of antioxidants of any fruit.
> 1/4 watermelon
> Lime
> Mint
> Sparkling mineral/soda water (optional)

Put the watermelon in the blender and whiz until it's a drink-able consistency. The seeds will stay a bit granular. Squeeze in a little lime juice. Serve room temperature or chilled with some torn fresh mint. Add sparkling mineral or soda water, if you like.

### 🕊 Apple and/or pear spritzer

**Serves 1**

> 1 lb (16oz/400g) of apples or pears, or a mixture
> 1-in (2.5cm) cube peeled ginger (optional)
> Sparking mineral water
> Sprig of mint (to garnish)

Juice the fruit. If you like ginger, juice the cube of peeled ginger with the fruit. Add the same amount of sparkling mineral water. Serve with a sprig of mint.

## The Store-cupboard

This includes items for all five biotypes – since you're bound to have lots of different sorts clamouring for food at some stage. Always buy organically grown foods, if possible.

**Breakfast cereals**
Plain, sugar-free cornflakes, puffed wheat, rice krispies, Weetabix
Kashi
Sugar-free, gluten-free muesli and muesli base

**Breads**
Wholemeal wheat
Rye
Pumpernickel
Vogel bread
Rice, barley, spelt, kamut, farro and naan breads

**Flour**
Stamp Collection All-Purpose Non-Wheat flour
Unbleached wheat flour, such as Shipton Mill

**Grains**
Brown rice
Whole-wheat
Whole oats and jumbo oats
Barley
Buckwheat (plain and roasted)
Millet
Maize
Spelt

Farro
Kamut
Quinoa
Yeast

**Pasta and noodles**
Whole-wheat, buckwheat,
    spelt, kamut, millet, rice,
    bean and vegetable flour
    pastas
Rice noodles

**Pulses**
Red, yellow and green
    lentils
Yellow and green split peas
Puy lentils
Dried beans

**Tinned goods**
Anchovies
Sardines
Tuna
Salmon
Baked beans, sugar-free
Chick peas,
Three-bean salad mix
    (cannellini, flageolet and
    aduki beans)
Tomatoes

**Condiments**
Olive oil
Balsamic vinegar
White wine vinegar
Sea salt
Black peppercorns

**Frozen fruit and vegetables**
Red berries
Blueberries
Raspberries
Redcurrants
Blackcurrants
Peas
Sweetcorn
Beans
Spinach
Cauliflower
Mixed vegetables
Broccoli

**Treats**
Green & Black Organic
    Chocolate, Toffee and
    Vanilla Ice-cream
Stamp Collection crisps

**Jars**
Barley malt extract
Black-strap molasses
Marmite

## Drinks

Café HAG (instant decaff)
Barley cup
Caro
Organic Coffee
Organic Tea (try Clipper varieties)
Decaffeinated organic coffee
Decaffeinated tea
Herbal teas
Biota vegetable juice
Norfolk Punch

## Snacks

Oatcakes
Brown rice cakes
Ryvita
Rye biscuits
Wallaby bars
Falafel

## Flavouring and seasonings

Fresh herbs and/or dried packet herbs
Schwartz's Italian seasoning
Peppercorns, black and white
Sea salt
Mild curry paste
Olive paste (tapenade)
Pesto

Anchovy paste
Tomato paste
Marmite
Vecon

## Spreads

Fresh peanut butter
Hazelnut spread
Cashew nut spread
Carob and nut spread
Sunflower seed spread
Tahini
Hummus
Fruit conserves made with fruit only and no added sugar

## Dips

Hummus
Guacamole
Tzatziki

## Sweeteners

Molasses (black–strap)
Molasses sugar
Muscovado sugar
Barley malt extract
Organic honey (Manuka, if possible)

## Butter and margarine

Butter, unsalted

Healthily produced
margarines, such as
Granose, Vitaquell and
Vitaseig
Olive oil spreads, such as
Biona

**Dairy produce**
Organic milk: cow's, goat's,
sheep's
Yoghurt: plain organic
cow's milk, Greek
sheep's milk, goat's milk

Cheese: sheep's and goat's,
both hard and soft
Soya milk ( Provamel,
Granose), soya cream
and cheese
Oat milk
Rice milk

**Miscellaneous**
Vegetable stock/bouillon
powder
Carob

# The Directory

Details are correct at the time of going to press, but as things do change, we can only apologise for any glitches.

## Complementary and alternative therapies

Please note: if you write to any of the following organisations, always enclose a large SAE.

Institute of Complementary
Medicine (ICM)
PO Box 194
London SE16 7QZ
Tel: 020 7237 5165
Website:
www.icmedicine.co.uk

The Aromatherapy
Organisations Council
PO Box 19834
London SE25 6WF
Tel: 020 8251 7912
Website: www.aoc.uk.net

The Bach Flower Centre
Mount Vernon
Sotwell
Wallingford
Oxon OX10 0PZ
Tel: 01491 834678
Website:
www.bachcentre.com
*For flower essences and infor-
mation about Bach Flower
Remedies.*

Biodanza UK
48 Clifford Avenue
London SW14 7BP
Tel: 020 8392 1433
E-mail:
   martello@biodanza.
   demon.co.uk
*Dance therapy centre that*
   *provides classes, training*
   *and information.*

Body Control Pilates
   Association
14 Neal's Yard
Covent Garden
London WC2H 9DP
Tel: 020 7379 3734
Website: www.body
   control.co.uk

Brahma Kumaris
65 Pound Lane
London NW10 2HH
Tel: 020 8727 3350
Website:
   www.bkwsu.org.uk
*Excellent site for meditation.*

The British Acupuncture
   Council
63 Jeddo Road
London W12 9HX

Tel: 020 8735 0400
Website: www.acupuncture.
   org.uk

The British Autogenic
   Society
Royal London
   Homoeopathic Hospital
Great Ormond Street
London WC1N 3HR
Website: www.autogenic-
   therapy.org.uk

British Chiropractic
   Association
Blagrave House
17 Blagrave Street
Reading
Berkshire RG1 1QB
Tel: 0118 950 5950
Website: www.chiropractic-
   uk.co.uk

The British Reflexology
   Association
Monks Orchard
Whitbourne
Worcester WR6 5RB
Tel: 01886 821207
Website:
   www.britreflex.co.uk

*For a list of practitioners, send
an SAE with a £2
cheque or postal order.*

British Wheel of Yoga
25 Jermyn Street
Sleaford
Lincolnshire NG34 7RU
Tel: 01529 306851
Website: www.bwy.org.uk

The Cranio-Sacral Therapy
   Association of the UK
Monomark House
27 Old Gloucester Street
London WC1N 3XX
Tel: 07000 784735
Website: www.craniosacral.
   co.uk

European Hellerwork
   Association
c/o Geri Harries
   (Hon. Sec.)
Thornfield
Stretton on Fosse
Moreton in the Marsh
Glos GL56 9RA
Tel: 01608 662848
Websites: www.heller
   work.co.uk or www.
   hellerworkeurope.com

Feldenkrais UK
East Holcombe
Shillingford
Tiverton
Devon EX16 9BR
Tel: 07000 785506
Website:
   www.feldenkrais.co.uk

General Council and
   Register of Naturopaths
2 Goswell Road
Street
Somerset BA16 0JG
Tel: 01458 840072
Website: www.naturopathy.
   org.uk

General Osteopathic
   Council
Osteopathy House
176 Tower Bridge Road
London SE1 3LU
Tel: 020 7357 6655
Website:
   www.osteopathy.org.uk

London School of T'ai chi
   chuan
PO Box 9836
London SE3 0ZG
Tel: 07626 914540
   (24-hour answerphone)

275

Website:
www.gn.apc.org/taichi

McTimoney Chiropractic
Association
21 High Street
Eynsham
Oxon OX29 4HE
Tel: 01865 880974
Website:
www.mctimoney.org.uk
*A gentle type of chiropractic.*

National Federation of
Spiritual Healers
Old Manor Farm Studio
Church Street
Sunbury on Thames
Middlesex TW16 6RG
Tel: 01932 783164
Website: www.nfsh.org.uk

National Institute of
Medical Herbalists
56 Longbrooke Street
Exeter
Devon EX4 6AH
Tel: 01392 426022
E-mail:
nimh@ukexeter.freeserve.
co.uk
Website: www.nimh.org.uk

The Reiki Alliance
27 Lavington Road
London W13 9NN
Tel: 020 8579 3813
Website: www.reiki
alliance.org.uk
*An international association
for highly qualified Reiki
masters only.*

Leigh Richmond
(aromatherapist)
The Life Centre
15 Edge Street
London W8 7PN
Tel: 020 7221 4602

The Society of
Homeopaths
4a Artizan Road
Northampton NN1 4HU
Tel: 01604 621400
Website: www.homeo
pathy-soh.org

Society of Teachers of the
Alexander Technique
129 Camden Mews
London NW1 9AH
Tel: 020 7284 3338
Website: www.stat.org.uk

The Sutherland Society
c/o 15a Church Street
Bradford upon Avon
Wiltshire BA15 1LN
Tel: 01225 868282
Website:
  www.cranial.org.uk
*For information on cranial
  osteopathy, and practitioners
  in the UK.*

UK Council for
  Psychotherapy
167–9 Great Portland Street
London W1W 5PF
Tel: 020 7436 3002
Website:
  www.psychotherapy.
  org.uk

*For information and contact
  details of qualified
  psychotherapists.*

European Hellerwork
  Association
c/o Geri Harries, Secretary
Thornfield
Stretton on Fosse
Moreton in the Marsh
Gloucestershire
GL56 9RA
Tel: 01608 662848
Website: www.heller
  workeurope.com
*An excellent contact for
  Rolfing in the UK.*

## Life coaching

We have been recommended a web-based organisation called
Life Coach UK at www.lifecoachuk.com, or (e-mail) info@
lifecoachuk.com. They have no telephone contact number.

Breakthrough Network for
  Work Life Coaching
29 Adine Road
London E13 8LL
Tel: 020 7473 5544
Website:
  www.lifeshift.co.uk

## Support and information

Alcoholics Anonymous
(AA)
UK helpline: 0845
7697555

Action Against Allergy
(AAA)
PO Box 278
Twickenham
Middlesex TW1 4QQ
Tel: 020 8892 2711

Allergy Research
Foundation
PO Box 18
Aylesbury
Bucks HP22 4XJ
Tel/Fax: 01296 655818
*A site for health professionals.*

Anaphylaxis Campaign
PO Box 275
Farnborough
Hants GU14 6SX
Tel: 01252 542029
E-mail:
anaphylaxis.campaign@
virgin.net
Website: www.ana
phylaxis.org.uk

British Allergy Foundation
Deepdene House
30 Belgrave Road
Welling
Kent DA16 3PY
Tel: 020 8303 8525
Fax: 020 8303 8792
Website: www.allergy
foundation.com

Hyperactive Children's
Support Group
71 Whyke Lane
Chichester PO19 2LD
Tel: 01243 551313
Fax: 01243 552019

Mission Possible
Website:
www.dorway.com/
possible.html
*International campaigners
against Aspartame.*

Narcotics Anonymous
UK service office: 020
7251 4007
UK helpline: 020 7730
0009

Seasonal Affective Disorder
  Association
PO Box 989
Steyning
BN44 3HG
Website: www.sada.org.uk

## Organic food and drink

Clipper Teas
Website: www.clipper-
  teas.com

Montesol Organic coffee
Website: www.great-
  coffee.co.uk

The Organic Gardening
  Catalogue
Riverdene Business Park
Molesey Road
Hersham
Surrey KT12 4RG
Tel: 01392 253666
Fax: 01932 252707
E-mail: chaseorg@aol.com
Website: www.organic
  catalog.com

Simply Organic Food
  Company

Tel: 0870 162 3010
Website: www.simply
  organic.net
*A nationwide delivery service
  for organic food.*

The Soil Association
Bristol House
40–56 Victoria Street
Bristol BS1 6BY
Tel: 0117 929 0661
Website: www.soil
  association.org
*A fantastic source of informa-
  tion on all aspects of
  organic food and living.
  They offer an organic directory, that provides details of
  every type of organic shopping, from box schemes to
  home delivery.*

## For Vegetarians and Vegans

The Vegetarian Society
Parkdale
Dunham Road
Altrincham
Cheshire WA14 4QG
Tel : 0161 925 2000
Fax: 0161 926 9182
E-mail: info@vegsoc.org
Website:www.vegsoc.org

The Vegan Society
Donald Watson House
7 Battle Road
St Leonards-on-Sea
East Sussex TN37 7AA
Tel:0845 458 8244
Fax: 01424 717 064
E-mail: info@vegan
    society.com
Website: www.vegan
    society.com

## Sources of nutritional supplements and natural health products

Ainsworths Homeopathic
    Pharmacy
36 New Cavendish Street
London W1G 8UF
Tel: 020 7935 5330
Website:
    www.ainsworths.com

Aroma1
E-mail: info@aroma1.com
Website: www.aroma1.com
*This US-based internet
    company has wonderful*

*organic essential oils, plus
lots of information.*

Biocare Ltd UK
Lakeside
140 Lifford Lane
Kings Norton
Birmingham, B30 3NU
Tel: 0121 433 3727
Fax: 0121 433 8705
E-mail:
    biocare@biocare.co.uk

Blackmores
The Naturopathic Health
  & Beauty Company Ltd
Willowtree Marina
West Quay Drive
Yeading,
Middlesex UB4 9T
Tel: 020 8842 3956
Email :
  blackmoresuk@intonet.
  co.uk
Website:
  blackmores.com.au
*For supplements and other
natural remedies.*

GNC (General Nutrition
  Centre)
Website: www.gnc.co.uk
*A useful website with both
products and information.*

The Healthy House
Cold Harbour
Ruscombe
Stroud
Glos GL6 6DA
Tel: 01453 752216
Fax: 01453 753533
E-mail: info@healthy-
  house.co.uk

Website: www.healthy-
  house.co.uk
*Mail-order company for water-
purifying equipment, light
boxes, eco-paints and a
wide variety of low-
allergen, environmentally
friendly and organic products.*

The Herb Society
Sulgrave Manor
Sulgrave
Banbury
Oxon OX17 2SD
Tel: 01295 768899
Fax: 01295 768069
E-mail:
  info@herbsociety.co.uk
Website:
  www.herbsociety.co.uk
*Information, links and prod-
ucts, as well as a quarterly
magazine,* Herbs.

Natural health products
Website: www.natural
  careweb.com
*A site devoted to sourcing all
aspects of natural health
products around the world.*

Neal's Yard Remedies
29 John Dalton Street
Manchester M2 6DS
Tel: 0161 831 7875
E-mail: mailorder@neals
yardremedies.com
Website: www.neals
yardremedies.com
*For aromatherapy essential
oils, herbs and herbal
products, homeopathic
remedies, flower essences
and much, much more.*

New Vistas Healthcare
Plassey Park
Limerick
Ireland
Tel: 00 35 3 61 334455
Fax: 00 35 3 61 331515
E-mail newvista@iol.ie
Website: www.newvistas
healthcare.com

Nutri Ltd
Buxton Road
New Mills
High Peak
Derbyshire SK22 3JU
Tel: 0800 212742
Fax: 0800 371371
E-mail: info@nutri.co.uk,
and orders@nutri.co.uk

The Organic Herb Trading
Company (formerly
Hambleden Herbs)
Court Farm
Milverton
Nr Taunton
Somerset TA4 1NF
Tel: 01823 401 205
Fax: 01823 401 001
E-mail: info@organicherb
trading.com
Website: www.organicherb
trading.com

Solgar Vitamins Ltd
Beggars Lane
Aldbury
Tring
Herts, HP23 5PT
Tel: 01442 890355
Fax: 01442 890366
E-mail:
simeoum@solgar.com
Website: www.solgar.com

Tanita Fat Monitors
c/o John Bell & Croydon,
50–54 Wigmore Street,
London W1U 2AU
Tel: 020 7935 5555
Fax: 020 7935 9605
E-mail: jbc@aah.co.uk

Website: www.johnbell
  croydon.co.uk

Viridian Nutrition
31 Alvis Way
Royal Oak
Daventry
Northants, NN11 5PG

Tel: 01327 878050
Website: www.viridian-
  nutrition.com
*Supplements and herbal
  products that are primarily
  organic, with no artificial
  additives.*

## Juicers

The Good Housekeeping Institute in London tested 8 juicers. Their top six centrifugal juicers in order of preference are:

Magimix Le Duo
Stockist information:
  01483 427411

Breville AWT Juice
  Extractor
Stockist: Argos, Tel: 0800
  525089
Website:
  www.argos.co.uk

Vitamine Juice Master
Stockist: Wholistic
  Research, Tel: 01707
  262686
Website: www.wholistic
  research.com

Philips Cucina HR1840
Stockist information:
  0845 601 0354
Website:
  www.philips.co.uk

Russell Hobbs 9919
Stockist information:
  0161 947 3170

Moulinex A7531P1
Stockist information:
  0121 202 0590
Website:
  www.moulinex.co.uk

283

## Rod and Sarah's choice

The juicer we use is the Kenwood JE600. It performs well but this model is in the process of being superseded by a bigger, better and slightly more expensive model (JE700).

Stockist information: 02392 476000

Website: www.kenwood.co.uk (not user-friendly, so perhaps try a store instead)

## More expensive juicers

The Champion Juicer

Oscar

Samson

These juicers may be available from your local stores, but if not try the contacts listed below.

Superjuicer
Stockist information:
0115 960 8646

The Green Life Juicer
Stockist information:
Cucina Direct, Tel:
0870 727 4300

## Useful websites

Website: www.savant-health.com
*A useful website for juicers (as well as nutritional supplements)*

Website: www.ferns nutrition.com
*Ships discount-rate juicers worldwide*

## Recommended reading

### Cookbooks

*River Café Cookbook Green*, by Rose Gray and Ruth Rogers (Ebury Press)

*The Complete Book of Food Combining*, by Kathryn Marsden (Piatkus Books)

*Real Cooking*, by Nigel Slater (Michael Joseph)

*Montignac Provencal Cookbook*, by Montignac Publishing

*The Detox Cook*, by Louisa J Walters, Aliza Baron Cohen and Adrian Mercuri (Kyle Cathie)

Any cookery book by Elizabeth David

Free recipes online: there are hundreds of free recipes available on the internet. Simply key in 'free recipes', press search, and take your pick.

---

### Music Therapy

*The Mozart Effect*, by Don Campbell (Hodder & Stoughton)
Available by mail-order from this shop which also stocks lots of other helpful products.

Presence and Presents
9 Brewers Lane
Richmond
Surrey TW9 1HH
Tel: 020 8332 6566

---

### Roderick Lane's choice

The books listed below have been pivotal in Roderick Lane's understanding of man and his dietary needs. As you can see, some are old and treasured friends.

*The New Cranks Recipe Book*, by Nadine Absensur (Phoenix)

*Dr Atkins Diet Revolution*, by Robert C. Atkins, MD (Bantam Books, 1972)

*Food Is Your Best Medicine*, by Henry G. Bieler, MD (Ballantine Books, 1965)

*The Glucose Revolution*, by Jennie Brand-Miller et al (Hodder & Stoughton, 1998)

*The Pulse Test of Allergy*, by Arthur F. Coca, MD (Max Parish, 1959)

*Cooking Without*, by Barbara Cousins (Thorsons, 1989)

*Overcoming Food Allergies*, by Gwynne H Davies, ND, MNTOS (Ashgrove Press, 1985)

*The Food and Mood Handbook*, by Amanda Gearing (Thorsons)

*Health via Food*, by William Howard Hay, MD (Harrap, 1934)

*The T-Factor Diet*, by Martin Katahan, PhD (Guild Publishing, 1989)

*Nutrition Almanac*, by Gayla J. Kirschmann (McGraw Hill, 1996)

*Eat Fat and Grow Slim*, by Richard MacKarness, MBBS (Harvill Press, 1958)

*Pritikin Program for Diet and Exercise*, by Nathan Pritikin and Patrick M. McGrady (Grosset & Dunlap, 1979)

*Tired or Toxic?*, by Sherry A. Rogers, MD (Prestige publishing, 1990)

*The Zone*, by Barry Sears, PhD (Regan Books, 1995)

*Atlas of Men*, by William H. Sheldon, PhD, MD (Gramercy, 1954)

## Juicing

*Juice High*, by Leslie Kenton and Russell Cronin (Vermilion)
*Superjuice*, by Michael van Straten (Mitchell Beazley, 2000)
*Juicing for Health*, by Caroline Wheater (Harper Collins, 1993)

## Magazines

*The Inside Story*
Berrydales Publishers
5 Lawn Road
London NW3 2XS
Tel: 020 7722 2866
Fax: 020 7722 7685
E-mail: info@inside-story.com
Website: www.inside-story.com
*A monthly subscription newsletter for allergy sufferers and anyone on a restricted diet.*

*What Doctors Don't Tell You*
2 Salisbury Road
London SW19 4EZ
Tel: 020 8944 9555
Fax: 020 8944 9888
E-mail: info@wddty.co.uk
Website: www.wddty.co.uk
*For news on medical issues, and publishers of several good books.*

The Food Magazine
94 White Lion Street
London N1 9PF
Tel: 020 7837 2250
*For news on food and food issues.*

# Index